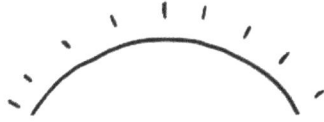

Soul Evolution

A Yogic Guide to the First Six Weeks After Birth

Yolande Hyde

Photographs by Ian Mathers

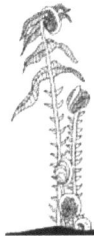

ISBN: 978-0-6454770-3-0

Dedication

The birth of my children was a watershed in my life.
It began a slow healing of the losses experienced in my own childhood, and it
gave way to the fullness and grace that loving another so completely can offer.

In this way love healed, and my children opened that door.
Each one in their own way.

Like all true healing, it wasn't always an easy path —
I suffered an ancestral cleansing that manifested as postnatal depression
with my first, a long overdue reckoning with my own mother in the second,
and challenges with the father of my children and the man
I loved with the third.

So what I offer among these pages has been felt and lived within me and, in
some quiet and slow-moving way, became a path of wholeness and healing.
My wish is that these words and gentle wisdoms give insight, understanding
and the nectar of shared experience to all who feel drawn to its message.
Yes, its Yoga, but it's also a whole lot more than that.

To this end I dedicate this book to the people who have been my life teachers
and who hold the essence of the very best of me:

Wiluna, Mahala & Elvis

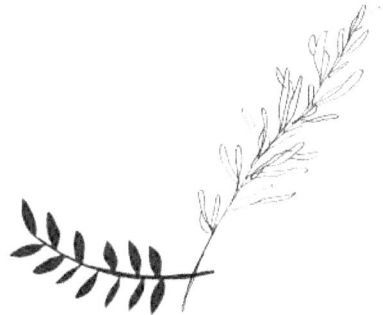

Contents

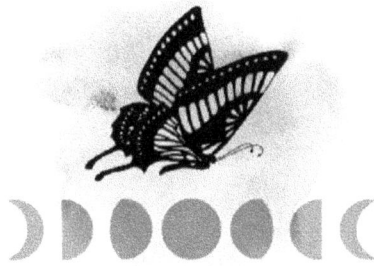

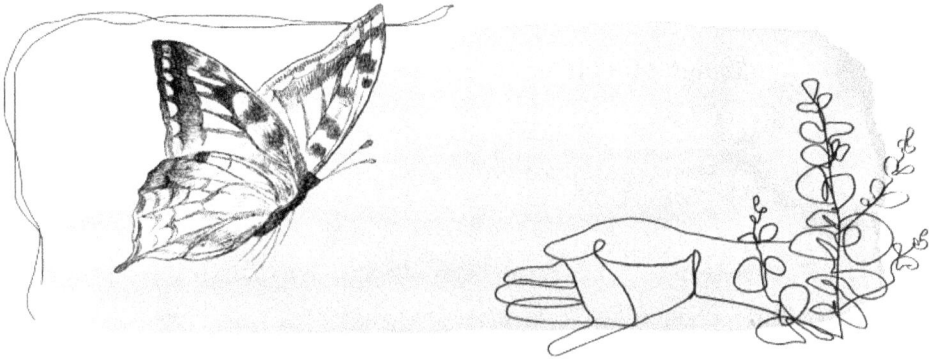

Some advice from mothers who have gone before....

The waters inside you are shifting to fit the newly created shape of the mother. They manifest themselves most obviously as the pure fluids of blood, milk and tears. The blood that follows the emptying of your womb, the milk that nourishes, bridges and bonds you to your child, and the tears that will fall as you move between the steady footing of what you know, and the vastness of this new world.

Expect that over the next six weeks you will be experiencing a myriad of physical and emotional readjustments as you align with your new Self. Use the practices contained in these pages to support your physical recovery and your emotional recalibration.See them as a medium for the spiritual growth and evolution of which becoming a mother is a pivotal part.

Deliveries come in all shapes and sizes, there's no reliable formula or pattern. If yours wasn't straight forward, for your body or your heart, or you don't feel ready to begin the yoga program straight away, forgive yourself. There aren't any rules for when to begin other than beginning where you are. The techniques given in this book are intended to support and nourish you in these tender times, not to become a chore or an effort.

If you were able to maintain an active pregnancy you will find returning to a yoga or movement practice quite a natural thing. However in some circumstances pregnancy can render exercise difficult, or even impossible. If that has been your experience it will be wise to pace yourself and move forward mindfully. As a general rule of thumb, seek advice on starting a yoga practice after any assisted delivery (inc forceps, vacuum or caesarean).

Gentle, concentrated movements are helpful in healing the soft tissue injuries that can result from birth. They do this by bringing healing blood and energy to the pelvic and lower back area, allowing passage to be free and open in the upper body, focusing your mind, and harnessing your own innate healing capacity. These sequences allow time to reflect and adjust to the changes your life is undergoing. In this way they also bring healing and a state of peace to the heart.

If any posture causes discomfort, increases your blood flow or affects your emotions negatively it is best to avoid or modify the practice. Seek the advice of your primary caregiver or a yoga teacher before beginning again.

In all cases take responsibility for yourself — listen to what feels good and what doesn't, and above all, follow these feelings and knowings with curiosity. Ask your wise mind — "Show me what it means to listen within."

"Keep your mind clear and your heart open
so that you can hear your truth"
—Teachings of Kuan Yin

Taking In

With great joy comes great pain.
With great love comes great fear.
The responsibility can feel tremendous.

Everything in your body is in recovery after the journey brought forward by pregnancy and birth. Depending on your delivery — fast or slow, vaginal or assisted, first baby or fifth — you have entered the period of 'taking in', and in so doing can plunge into every emotion possible, sometimes all in one day. You are recalibrating and redefining the person you are with this wonderful new being in your life.

Your body will be experiencing the bruising, aching and bleeding. It happens during those first tender nights and the coming of your milk. Your heart may be carrying an unbearable love, an unsettling doubt, anxiety or an unexplainable sense of connection and homecoming. Somehow all of this must be 'taken in; understood, compassionately accepted or lovingly let go.

There are six practices in this book and this first one is to support that 'taking in' process through all the levels of your Mother being: physical, emotional and spiritual. It isn't about losing weight or toning muscles, it's only goal is to welcome you back into your body. You are growing and changing daily as you go about learning all the gentle things required to feed your baby, comfort another and be present in this new way.

Let your yoga be a soft and kind thing in your life.
Practice daily.

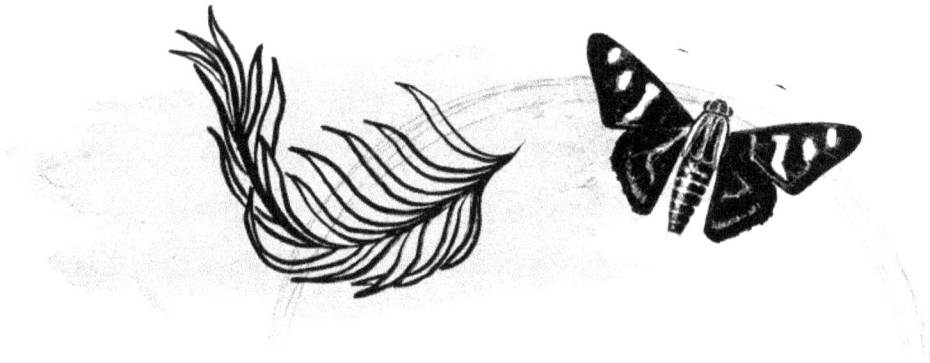

Welcome home. This is a whole new You:

You can't access the necessary wisdom through the external world, nor will you find value through possession or inheritance. The only space from which you can really view your new Self is from behind your own eyes. So once you feel comfortable in the postures let them close....

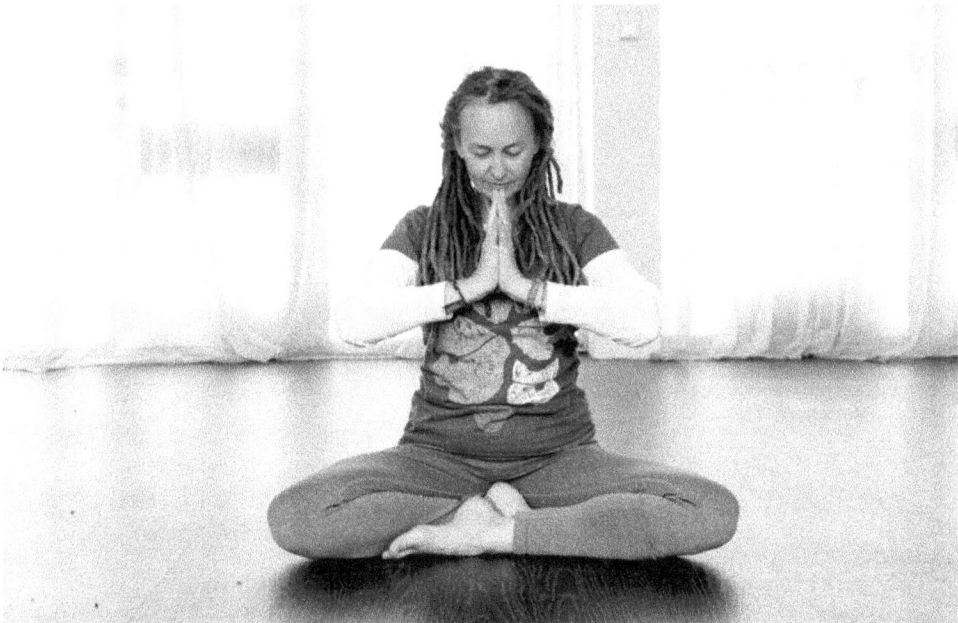

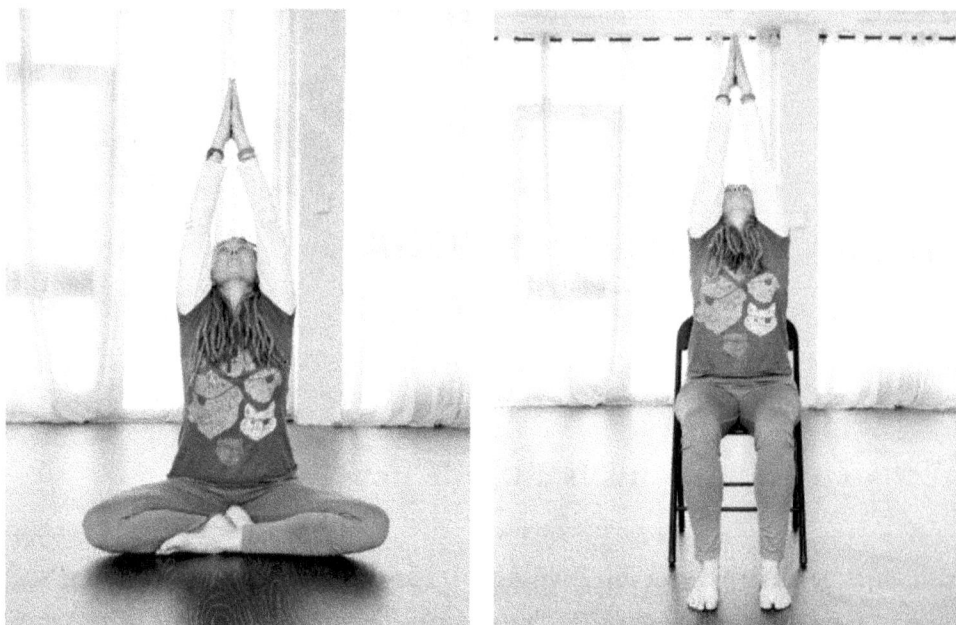

From an easy cross-leg position or from your chair, gently extend your arms to the sides of the body, place your fingertips on the floor.

Inhale and raise the arms over your head bringing the palms of your hands together in prayer.

Exhale and lower the hands following your centre line. Take the arms and the exhalation past the heart and belly till the fingertips come apart and return to the starting position with fingertips to the floor.

Repeat 2 – 8 times.

Opening the container:

Coming into a practice like yoga for the first time after such a big experience is like driving a new car. Everything is in a slightly different place, the driver's vista has changed and the engine has an unfamiliar revolution. Start gently, get to know yourself again, this is just the beginning.

i) Neck release

These can be done in the order given or as a stand alone.

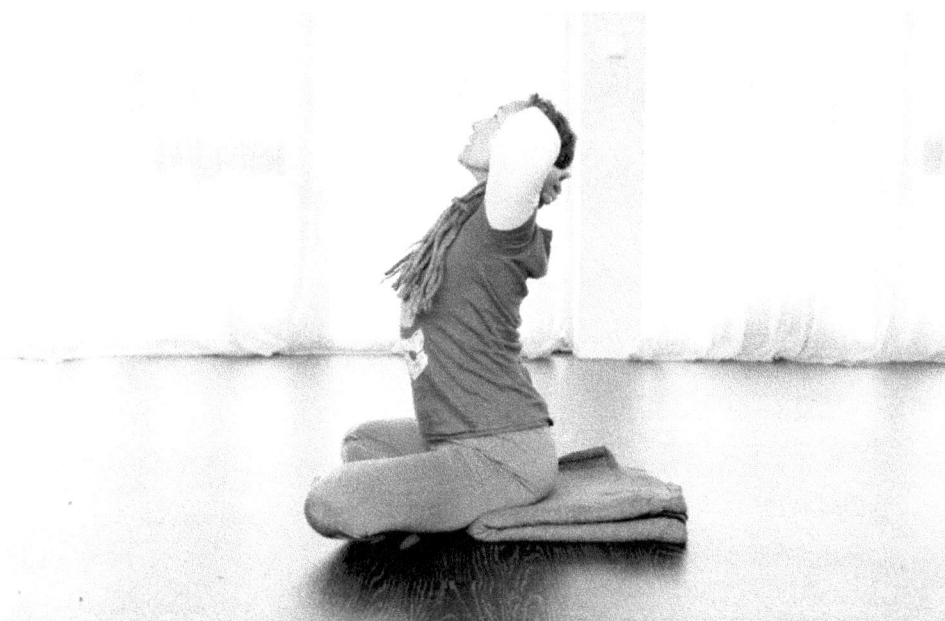

From your seated position, interlace the hands at the back of the neck, elbows wide. Inhale, open the elbows wider, broadening the chest, and let the head drop back a little to look towards the ceiling, feeling the throat, inner arms and chest.

Exhale, squeeze the elbows together, drop the chin to the collarbones and look towards the belly. Open the neck and upper back.

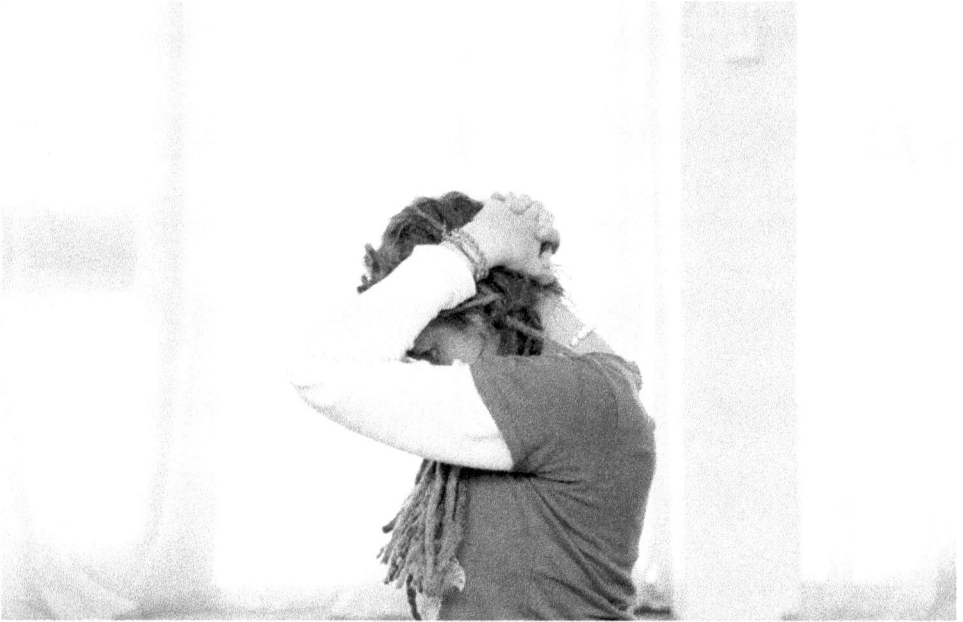

Repeat 4 – 6 times slowly with the breath.

ii) Sides of the body

Keeping the left hand where it is behind the neck, place the right hand on the mat in line with the right hip. Look along the top elbow if the neck permits.

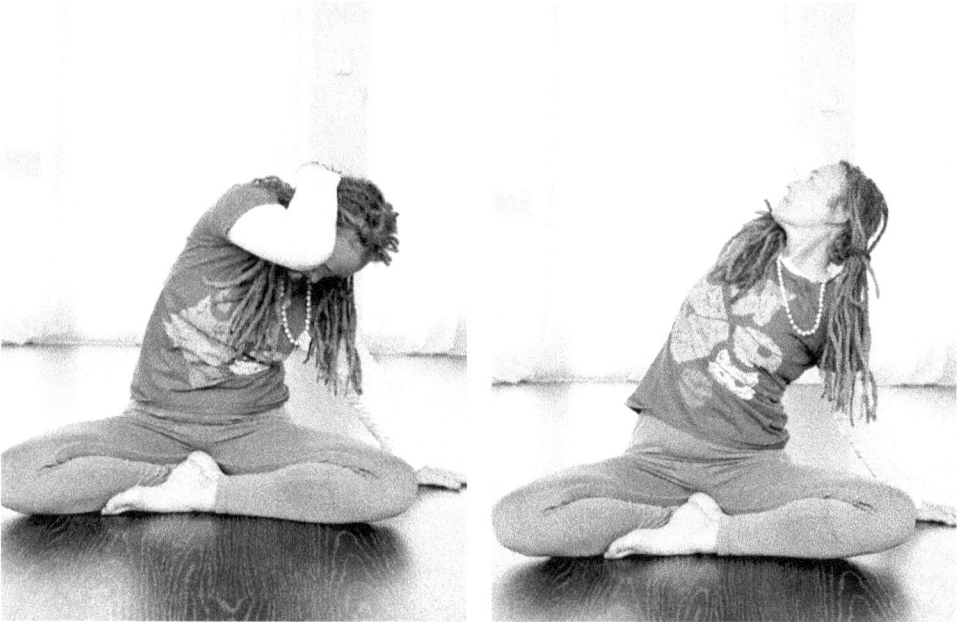

Inhale, roll the left elbow back, and open the chest

Exhale, roll the left elbow and rib cage forward moving just enough to feel the sides.

Repeat 2 – 3 times each side.

iii) Shoulder opener

Change the cross of the legs.

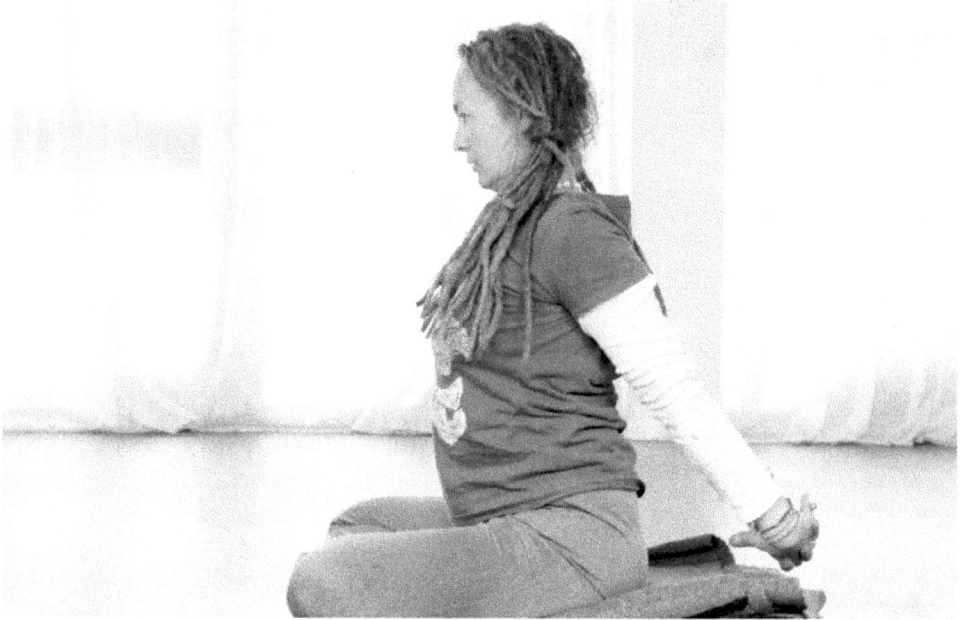

A) Interlace the hands at the sacral area, drop the knuckles to the floor, squeezing the shoulder blades together. Look up.

Inhale, press the chest forward and open. Lengthen the arms.

Exhale, raise the arms a little higher ifcomfortable. Depress the shoulder blades — if comfortable.

B) Release the arms. Interlace them in front of your heart, turning the palms away.

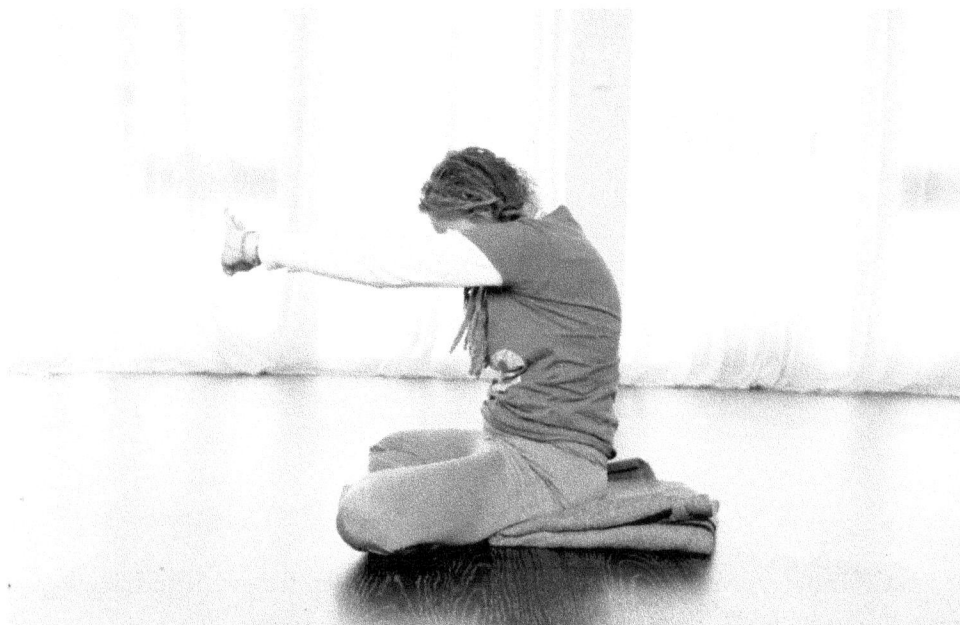

Exhale, and draw the chin inwards as you open into the upper back area. Let the spine curve towards the wall behind you and open as the chest gently rounds in on itself.

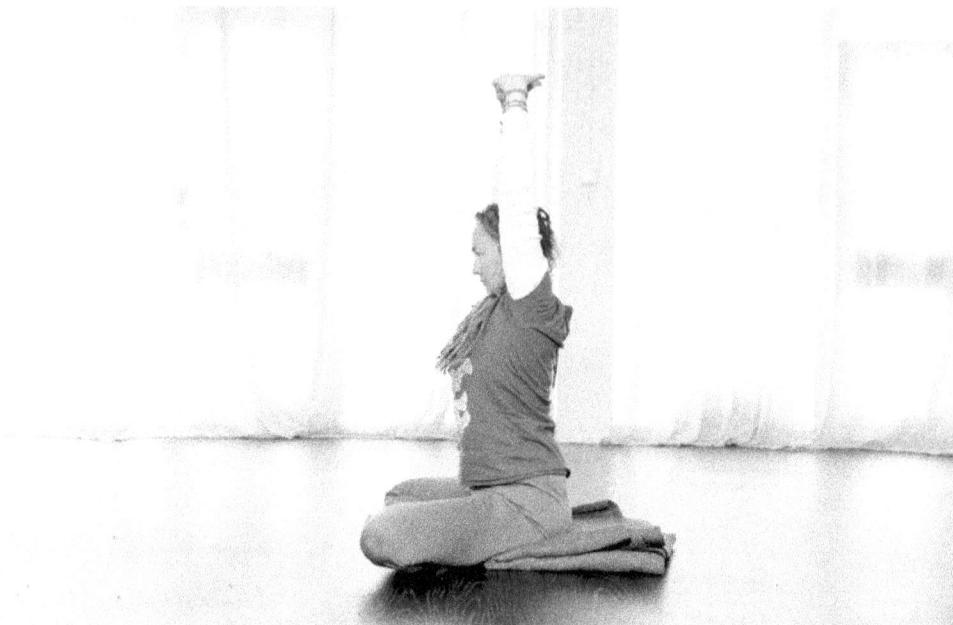

C) Inhale, raise the arms above the head with fingers interlaced and palms facing the ceiling. You may be able to align the upper arms with the ears or your arms may sit more forward than this. Both work. Take a few breaths. Lengthen the sides.

Exhale. Release and return to A).

Repeat cycle 3 – 4 times.

Taking a still point. **Seated Forward fold:**

Folding forward into yourself helps you lean into the quiet places that might otherwise be unheard. To do this invites the potency of a candle flame that serves to reset your light.

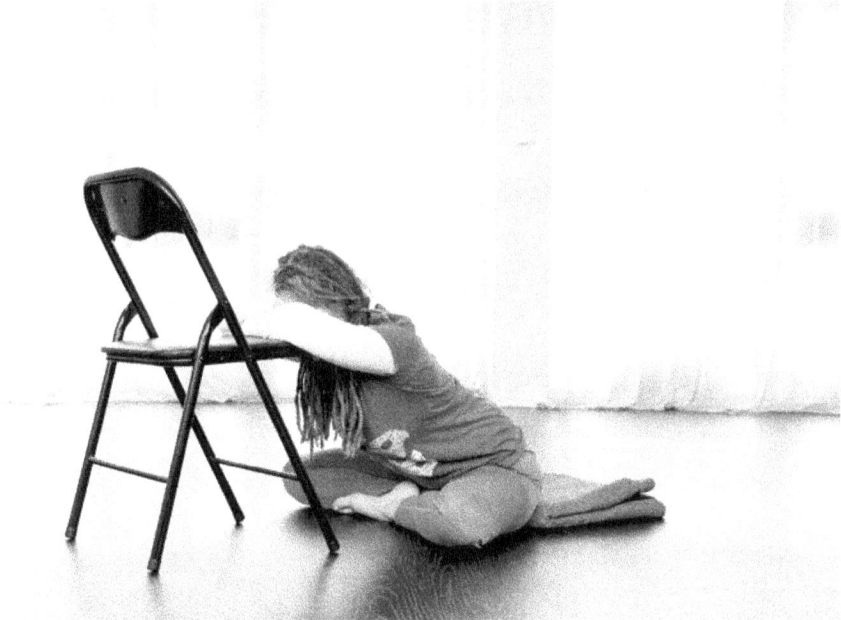

From your easy-cross position or chair, allow yourself to fold forward towards the floor or a support like a chair or sofa. Feel your hips, lower back and sacral area gently opening. Walk the torso to the right, allowing the left ribcage to roll a little towards the floor. Take a few breaths into the space that is created. Repeat to the left.

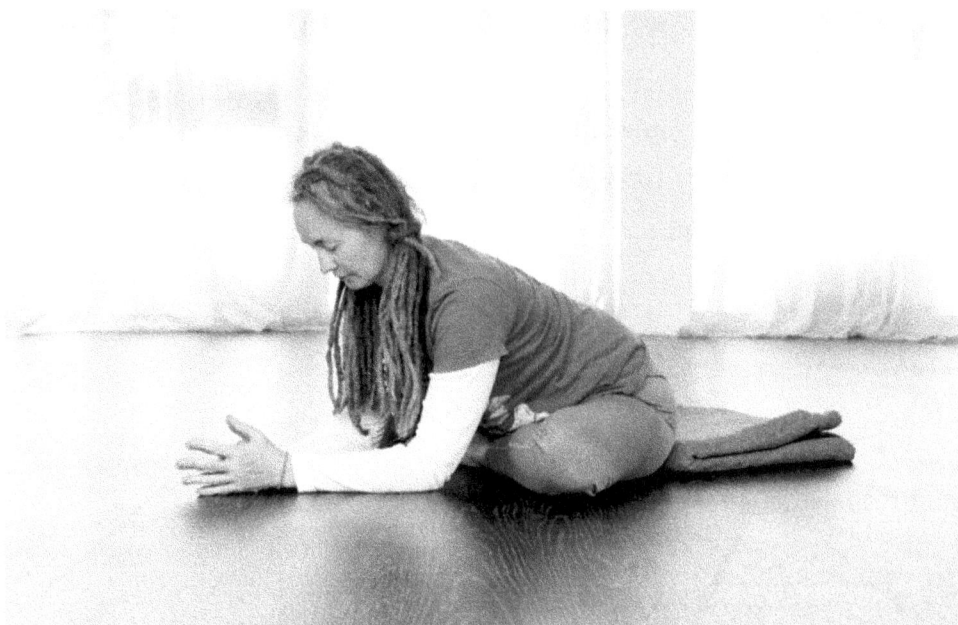

Return to the centre, bring a support under your forehead so you can rest — a cushion, chair or yoga block. Take 8 – 10 smooth breaths here, allowing your belly to be absolutely soft in its surrender. Try to be here in your comfortable darkness with compassion and acceptance for whatever you see or feel.

Change the cross of the legs and repeat on the opposite side.

Feeling the current. **Jatari Parivrtta (supine twist):**

The spine is like a superhighway for your nerve impulses, your consciousness and is what tethers you to the divine. To move, hydrate and massage its spaces means to open to the ocean of this potential.

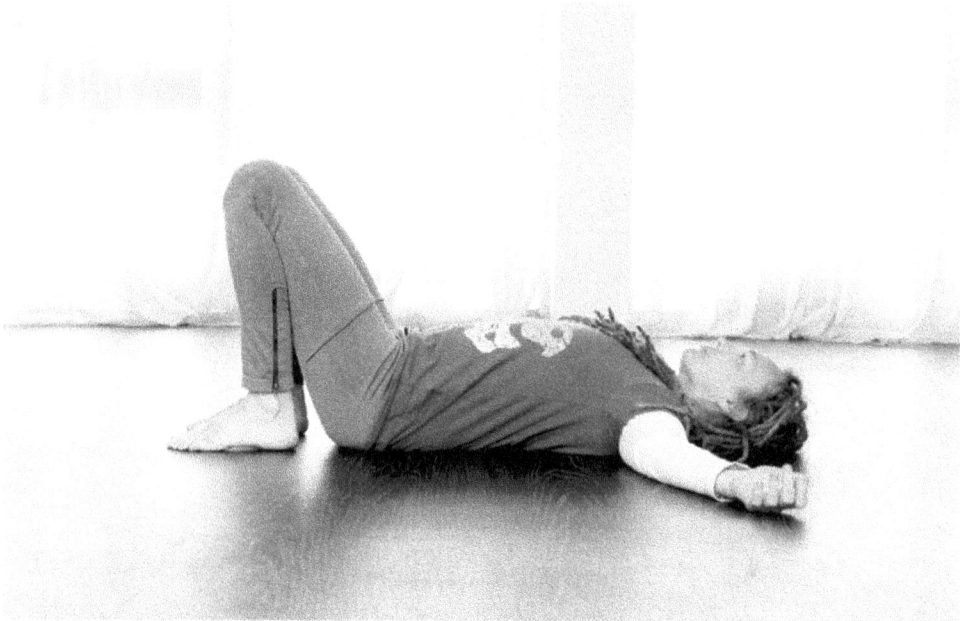

Come to lying on the floor on your back. Have the knees bent and the feet on the floor at shoulder width. Extend the arms, placing the hands just beside the hips (or at shoulder height for a deeper chest stretch).

Exhale, drop the knees to the right, look to the left.

Inhale, centre, and repeat smoothly from side to side, 4– 8 times.

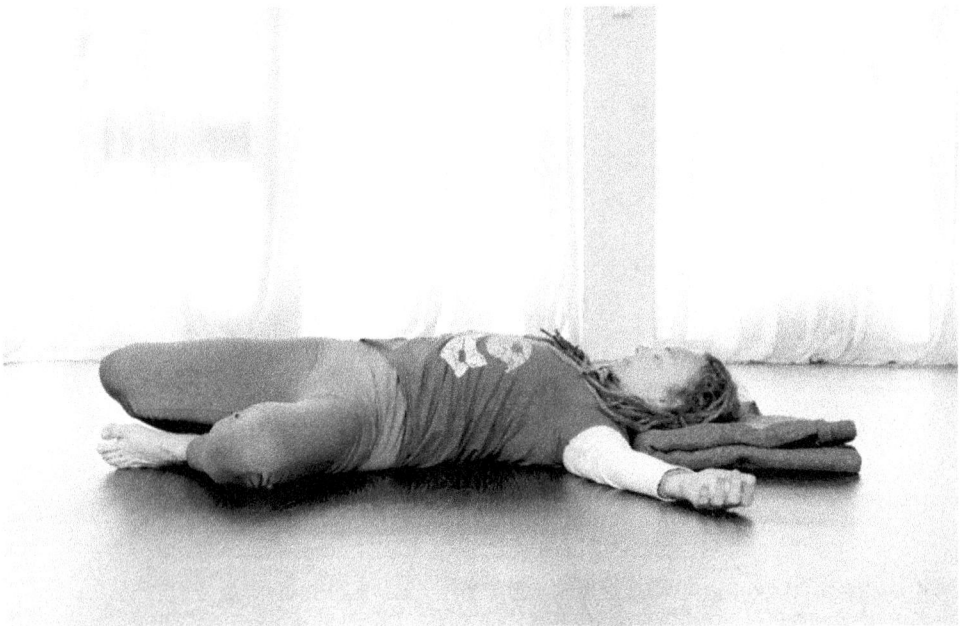

Hug the knees in towards the chest to finish. Let your belly drop back into your body and the back fall symmetrically to the floor supported. Stay here for as long as needed.

Finding your ground.

Nadi Shodhana (Alternate Nostril breath):

The breathing practices are the touchstone for a mother's sanity and steadiness in uncertain times. Completely portable, quick and effective, and so very simple. This is now the practice to cultivate and prioritize above all others.

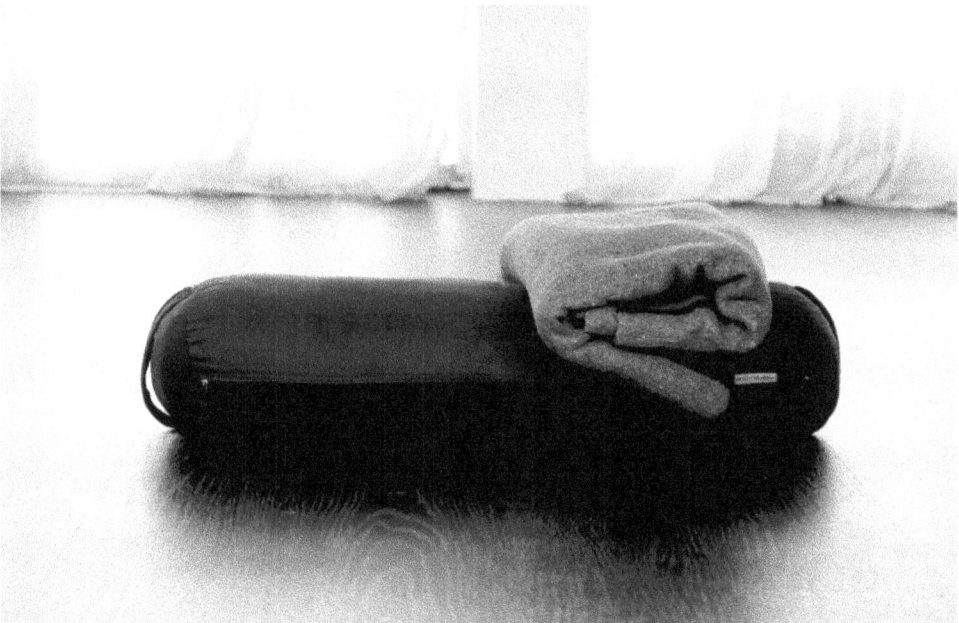

Re-adjust yourself for a supported breathing practice by folding a blanket or towel to form a low spinal support.

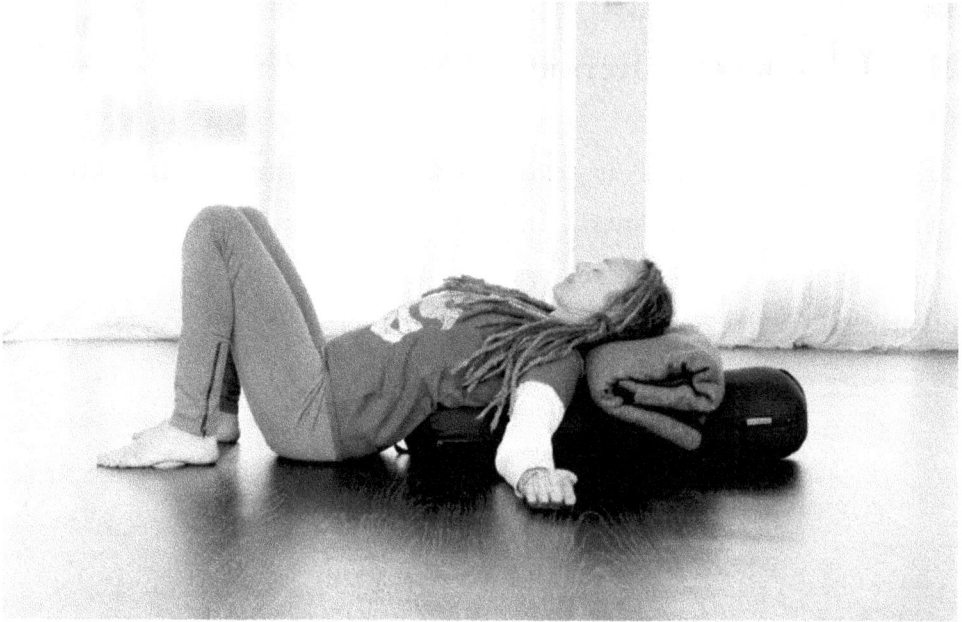

With your buttocks on the floor just in front of the support, lay your spine down over its length, creating a gentle rise and space for the ribs to fall a little either side. Ensure your head is supported with the chin resting a little way towards your breastbone. You can have your legs out long, in an easy cross shape or knees bent with feet on the floor. It should feel good. Adjust until it does.

The technique

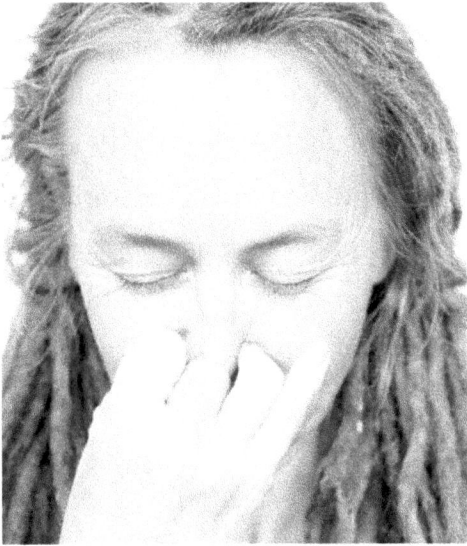

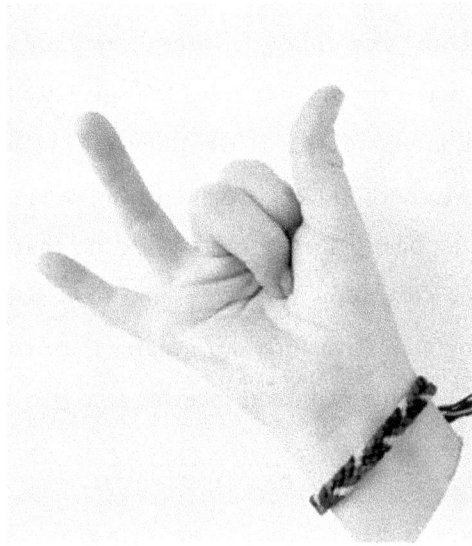

1. Holding your right hand in front of your face, begin by placing the thumb to the flesh of the right nostril and the ring finger to the flesh of the left nostril. Either drop the index and ring finger to your third eye space or fold them into your palm.

2. Close the left nostril and inhale slowly and deeply through your right nostril.

3. Now close off the right nostril, open your left and exhale completely.

4. Keep the left nostril open and inhale fully.

5. Close the left, open the right and exhale.

This completes one round of alternate nostril breathing. Set a timer for 3 – 5 minutes and practice with complete focus on the alternating current of breath.

Integrate yourself. **Savasana:**

Don't skip this. It consolidates your work and represents the most important phase of the practice. It's easy to feel compelled to be busy, a badge of honour we wear to define our value and our purpose. Here in the early rise of Motherhood, we are redefining the expression of who we are in the world, and the best place from which to do that is steeped in our own quiet. Listen and be still, allow the expression of your old Self to give way, you are surrounded by a creative force far greater than you know. We need only be still and wait. Our only task is to receive.

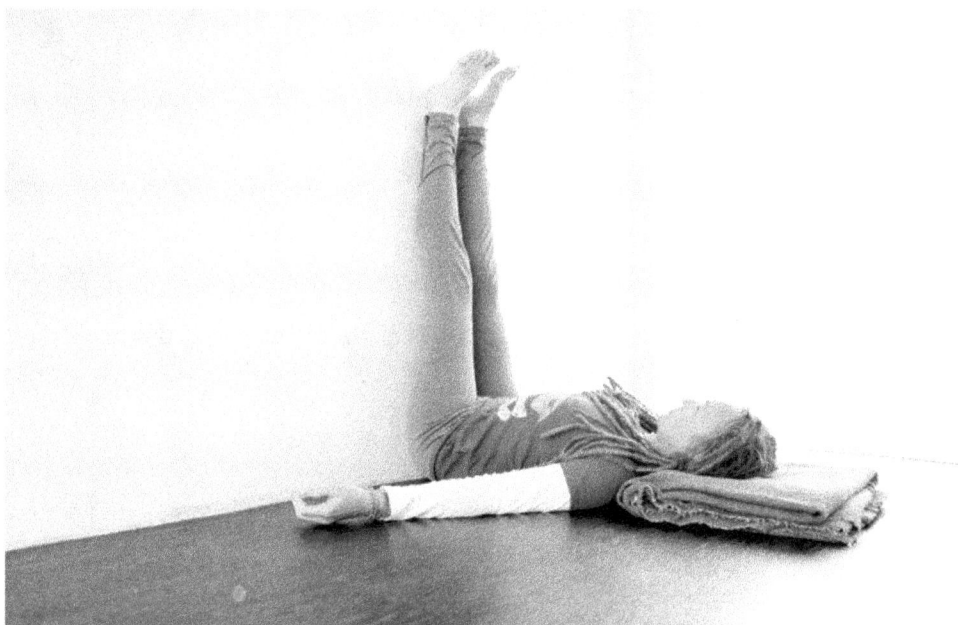

A beautiful way to do this is with a Legs-up-the-wall position. Draw a support under the lumbar spine and one under the neck. Alternatively lay yourself out flat on your back on the floor with a support under the backs of your knees. Cover your eyes with an eye wrap or eye bag and give yourself permission to sink into a quiet and still place. This is where the real work happens.

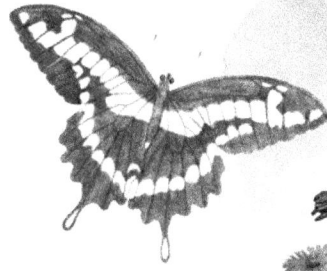

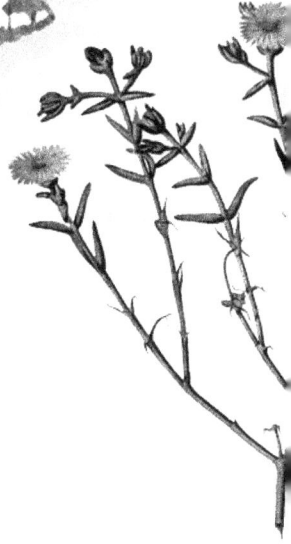

Taking Apart

Flesh of your flesh. Bones of your bones.

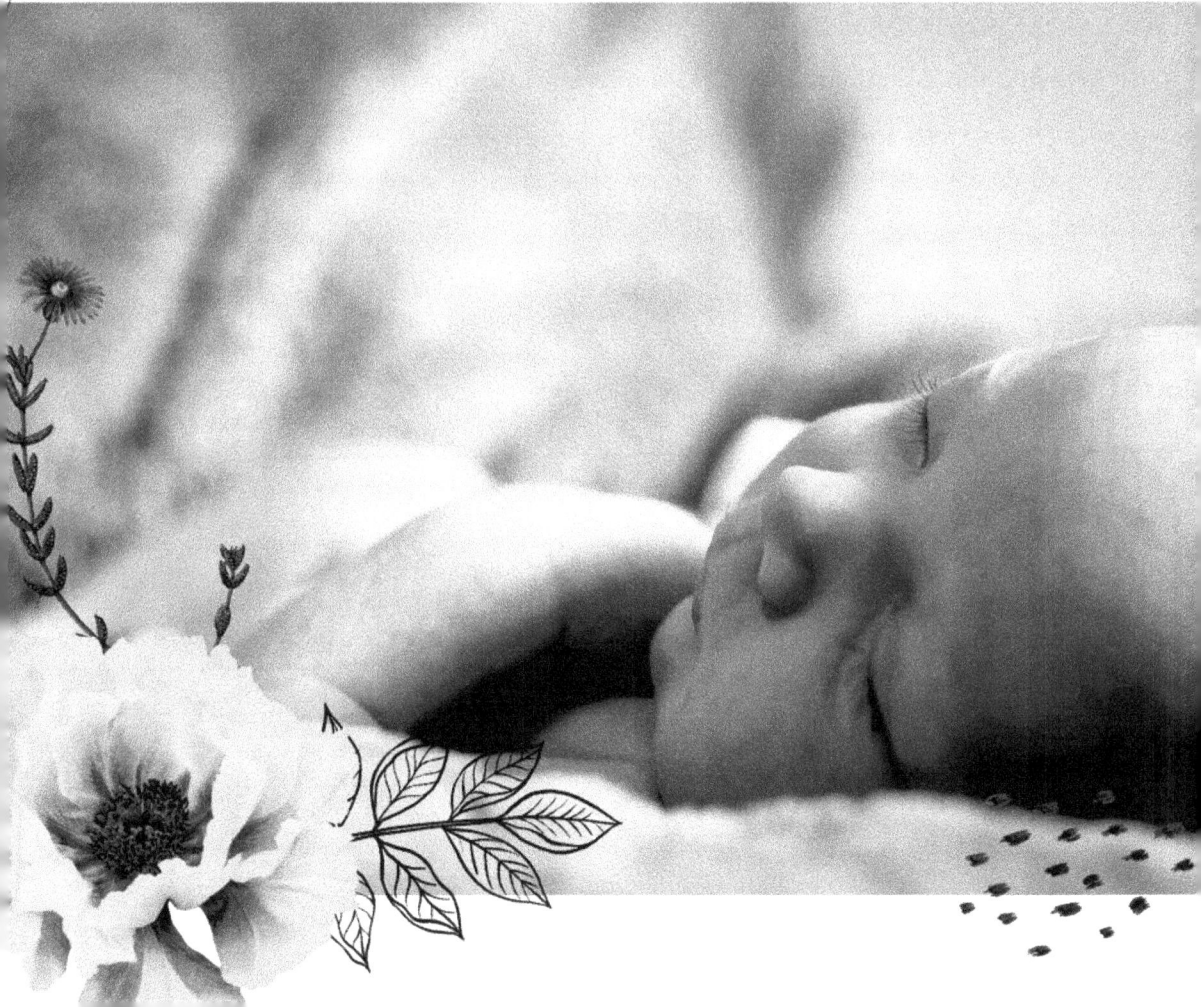

In this second week your body is transitioning from a hormonal high to the real work. You start developing the balance of giving and receiving through your milk and feeling forward into new life rhythms — feeding, sleeping and falling in love. You can sense the healing happening in your physical body, as your blood strengthens and your immediate wounds heal. Though you feel the sunlight you may also be falling at the feet of a deep emotional process.

Dear Heart, you've got this. Keep yourself and your baby protected from overstimulation and the chaos of the outside world for as long as you can. Explore the deep pool of each other and let others mother you. Life won't always be like this; your job now is to surrender and integrate what has just happened as best you can and not to feel the responsibility of housework or the demands of others.

Concern about this vulnerable little one, and the tremendous wonder and responsibility can be unsettling. Lean into the grounding and stabilizing support of those around you, lean into the practice on these pages, lean into all the tools you have gathered that have brought you to this moment. Talk to your midwife or compassionate other if it feels overwhelming, but above all remember, you were born for this.

Tell your story. It's what we do as women. ask questions and, in your quiet moments. use your silence to integrate this experience deep into your heart. and see its beauty and your strength in the face of it.

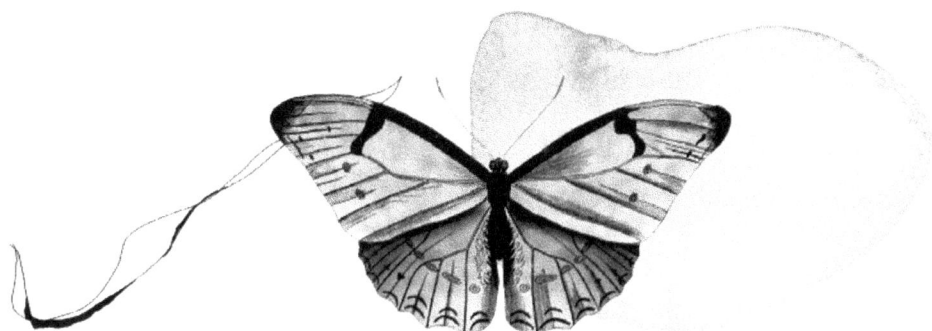

Return home. **Seated practice:**

This second practice stays low to the ground to hold you steady while it invites you to explore a little of your returning strength. As always, approach each posture as if it's brand new. Listen to your body for signs and clues that all is well, and as you gain familiarity with it over the week let it comfort the parts of you that feel less sure.

Let's begin in your seated pose just as you did last week. Use these few minutes to be with yourself in silence. Watch your breath rise and fall. Cast your eye over your internal world. Smile or cry. You are beautiful either way.

Everytime you come to this place it will be different. Take strength from that. You are changing and growing and learning and loving. These are precious days indeed.

Find your centre. **Cat cow and its variations:**

When things change fast, learning a technique to bring you back to your centre is a life raft. If your emotional centre feels too close or scary or unknowable, start here with your physical centre and work inwards from that peripheral understanding.

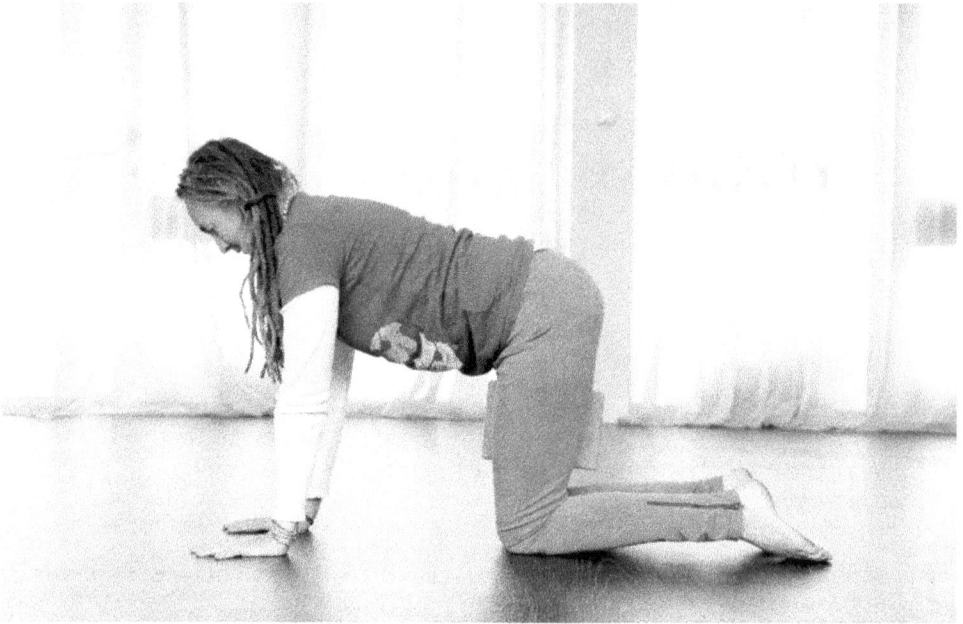

(i) Coming to an all-fours position with hands under your shoulders, fingers spread wide, and knees under your hips. I have added a yoga block between the middle of the thigh bones here. It is optional, however, it can be very supportive if the lower back is tender or sore.

Inhale, look up, open the chest through the upper arms and lift the tailbone to the ceiling. Let the belly gently stretch from pubic bone to throat.

Exhale, draw the belly back a little into the spine, tuck the chin under to open the neck and curl the tailbone under.

Repeat smoothly with even breaths 8 – 10 times.

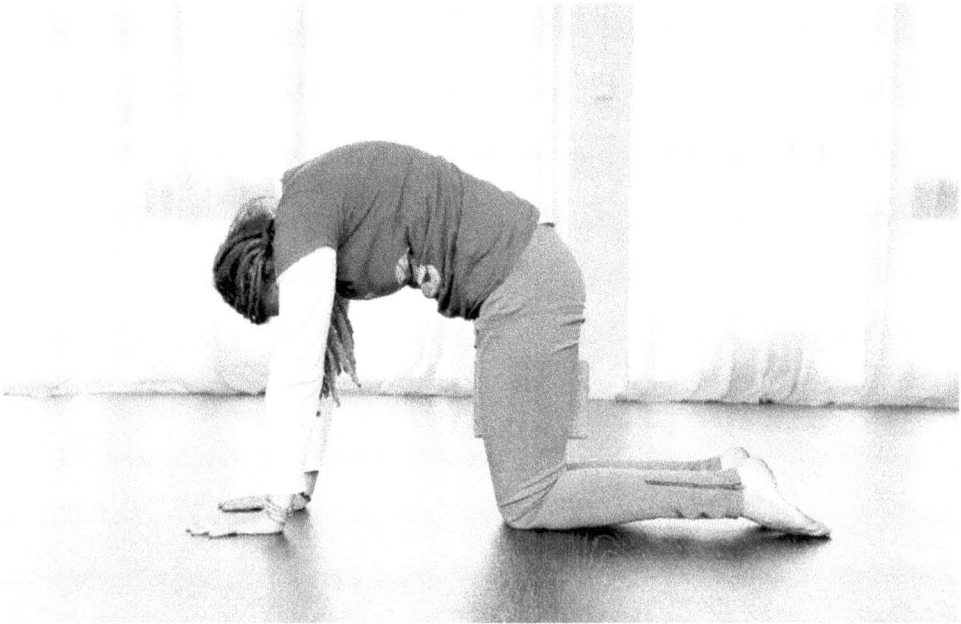

(ii) While continuing your breath and movement flow, let the shape change. Now imagine you are moving your outer ribs around the inside rim of a hula hoop — to the right, beneath you, to the left, to the ceiling. Keep your breath even and send it into all the opening spaces you can feel.

Keep working with this for as long as it feels good. Be sure to change direction.

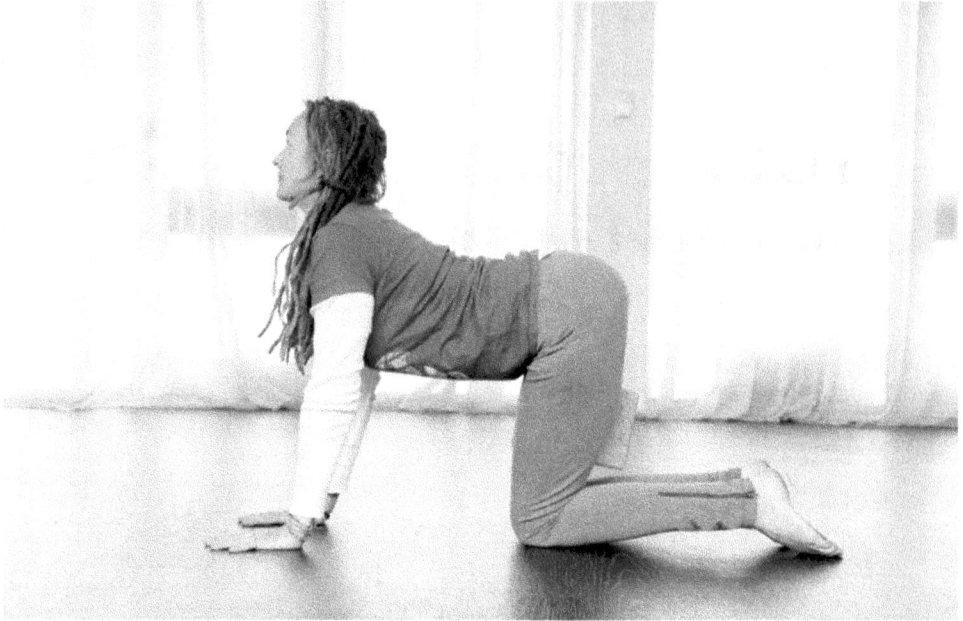

(iii) Exhale, arch the spine to the ceiling and roll the buttocks back towards the heels until they are resting and you are in child's pose. Have the hands extended forward or elbows bent, forehead on the floor or resting on a folded blanket or yoga block.

Take a few breaths here and feel the softness of your centre as you step inwards.

Taking stock of what's behind you.
Salabhasana (Locust) and its variations:

The back body holds life's greatest mysteries. It is a part of ourselves we will never actually see, an unknown perspective yet one that is critical to our upright self and our forward movement. It holds the energy of the past and the percussive press of the urge to move forward. Arriving here acknowledges what we have come from, and illuminates who we are becoming. YES!

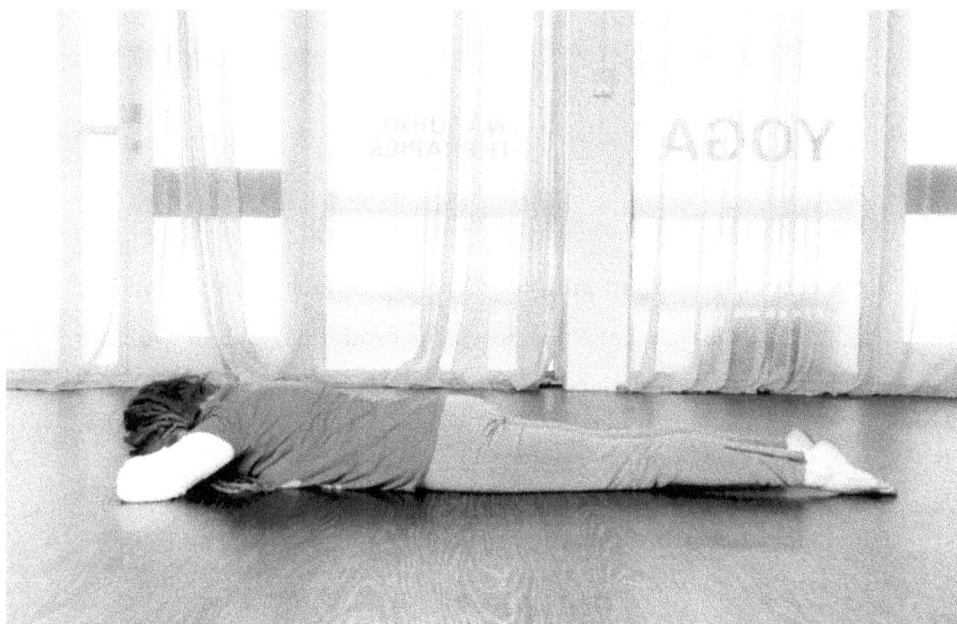

Come to lie on your belly, elbows bent, and rest the forehead on the backs of the hands. This can feel foreign at first but the floor can serve to gently press the organs in and up if it's comfortable. Legs extended behind you at hip width or wider. Gently move the pubic bone up towards the navel, feel it move into the floor with the lower spine and buttocks firm. Make the legs strong by pressing down the tops of the feet.

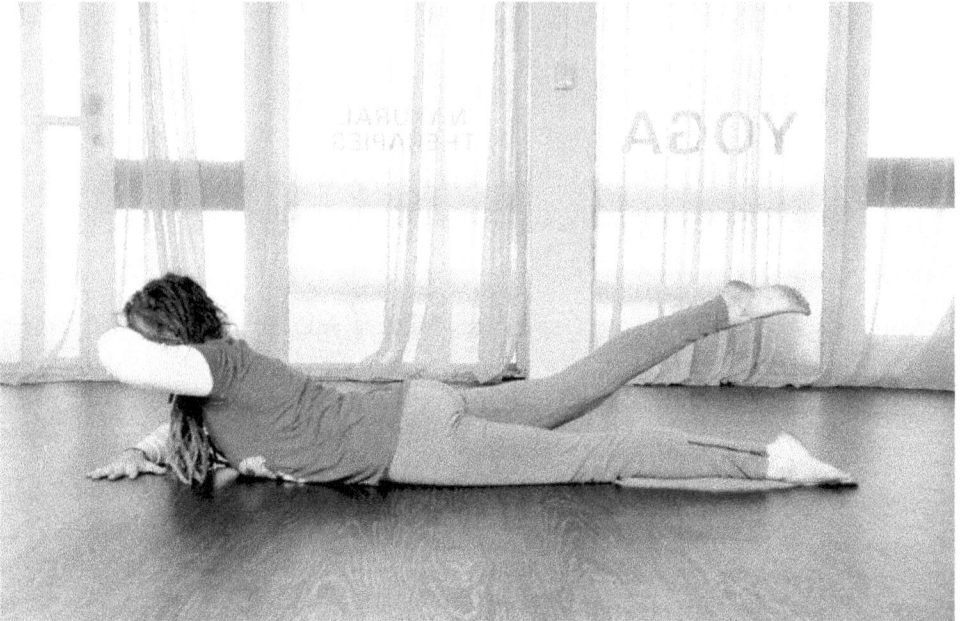

Exhale, raise the torso and keep the right back-of-hand on the forehead while you keep the left arm grounded and supporting the lift a little. At the same time raise the left leg. Feel the diagonal in the back.

Inhale and lower both to the ground.

Exhale, raise the left arm and the right leg, repeating on the opposite side.

Repeat, alternating 4 – 8 times.

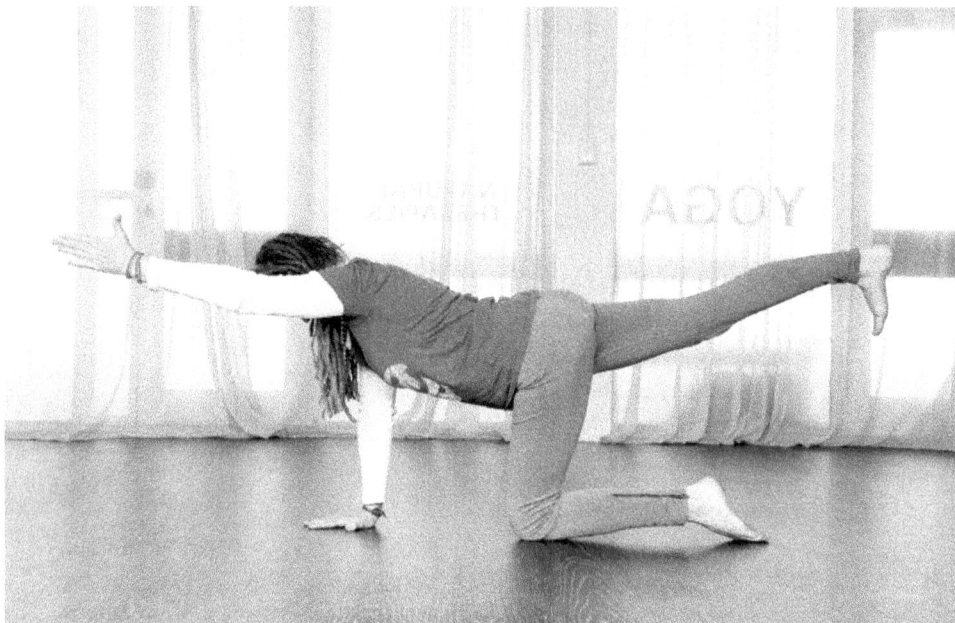

*If lying on your belly causes discomfort in your breasts or anywhere else the position can be done from all fours following the same directions but with the raised arm extended in line with the shoulder.

Release into what is. **Floor twist variation:**

To tone then soften is the medicine of the heart as it gives away and receives in a perfect balance of contract and release. The effects of the contraction in the previous pose can be sweetly countered and used to find softness and balance in the release of this floor-based twist. Look for absolute surrender.

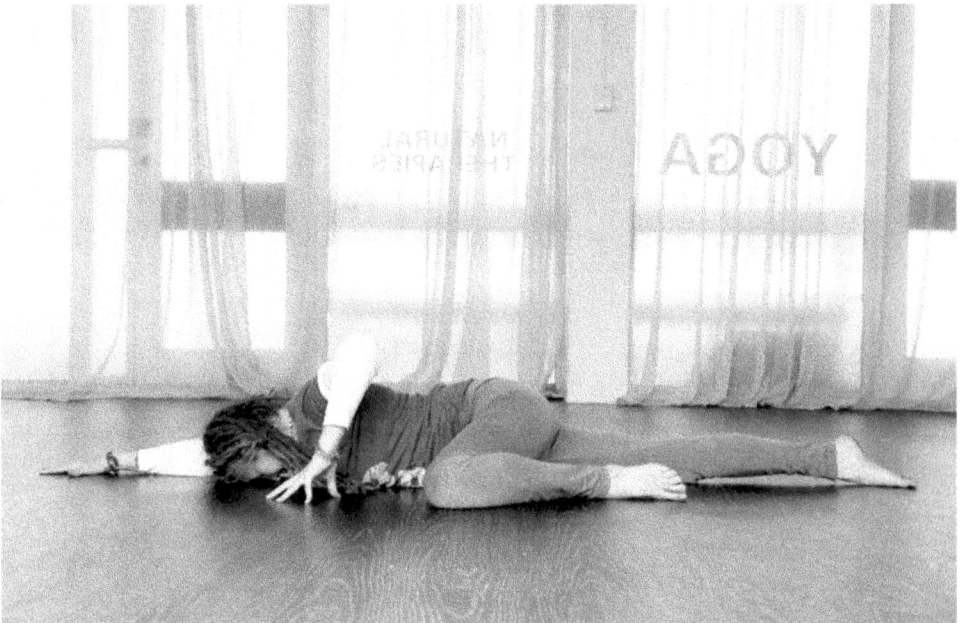

From your face-down position draw the right hand in under your right shoulder as a support. Draw the right knee up so that you can look down and into it. Extend the left arm along the floor at 12 o' clock.

Exhale, raise the right arm up towards the ceiling and drop it over to the floor behind you, allowing the body to follow and only going as far as feels comfortable.

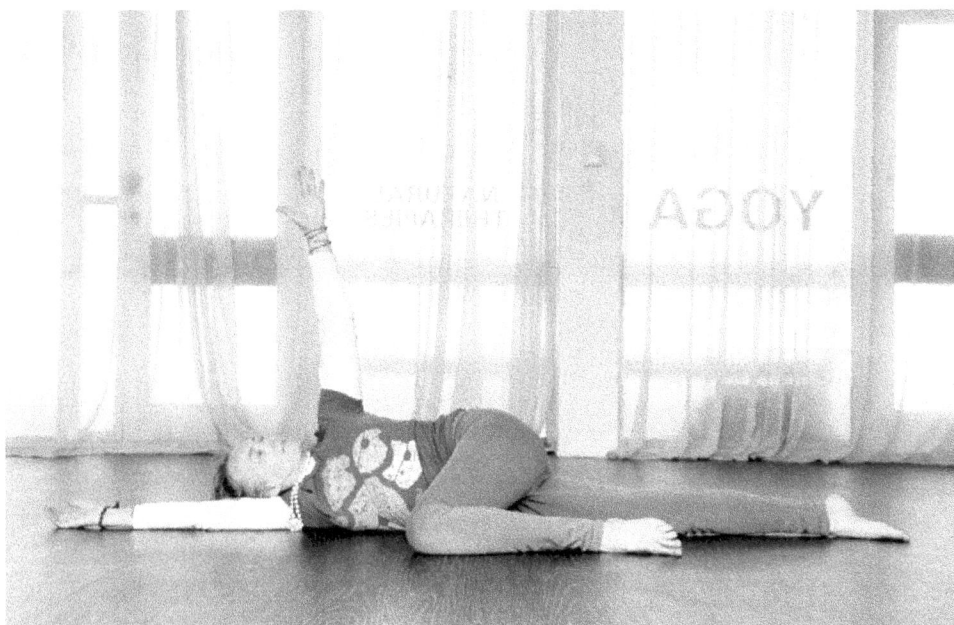

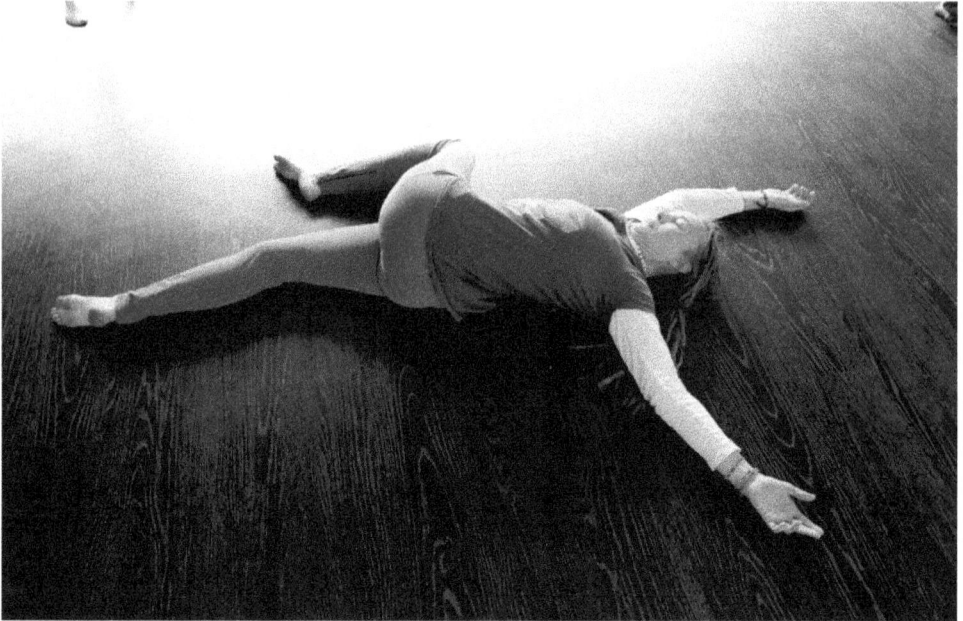

Keep reaching back until you anchor the shoulder blades and feel the sweet spaces between your bones. Allow yourself a few breaths here while everything seeks gravity. Try to relax — even your buttocks. If this is difficult or feels restrictive, focus on grounding your shoulder blades and add a cushion or yoga block support under the bent knee and shin bone.

Inhale, and return to your belly.

Exhale, and repeat on the opposite side.

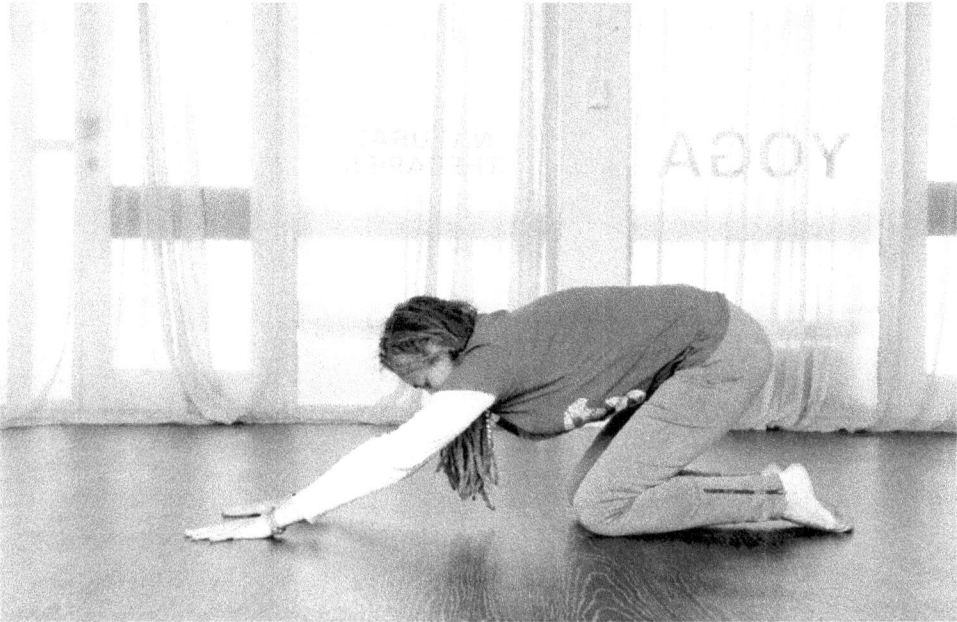

Returning to the centre, press the chest up using the hands and round the buttocks back to child's pose as you did before. Take a few breaths here and feel the press of your belly to the thighs and the doming of your back with the breath. After a few breaths, widen the knees to the width of the mat.

Sink. All is well.

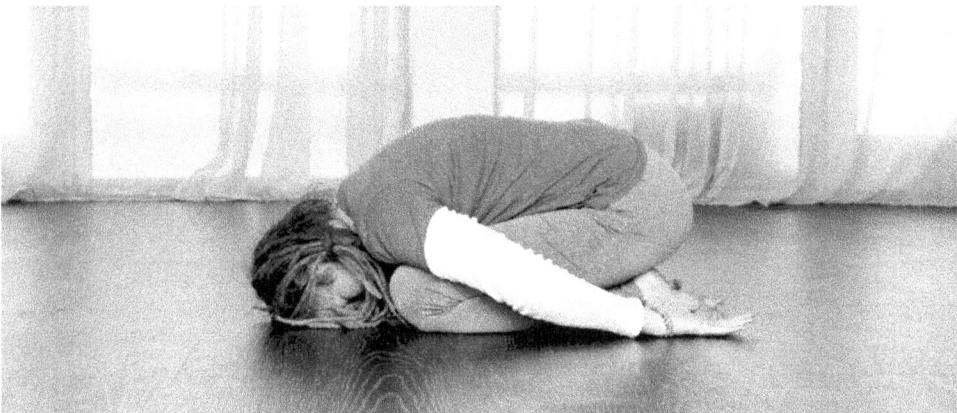

Quieten the mind.

Restore the senses: Siddhasana (Easy cross-leg):

This is the moment of return. How we feel when we return can help us gauge the effectiveness of the practice on any given day.

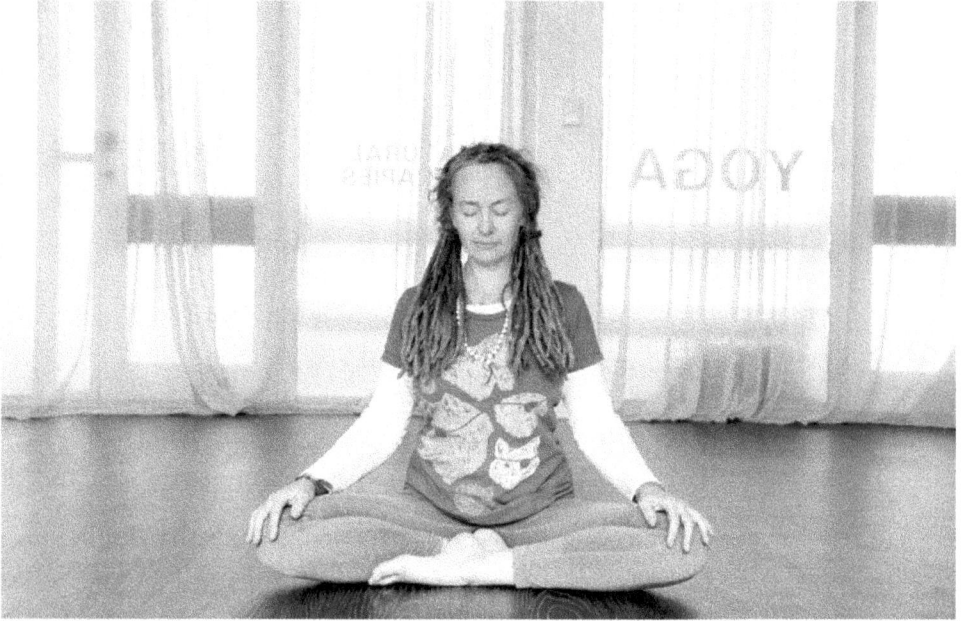

Come back to your easy cross-leg or chair for a seated base. Use this time to either sit quietly in your silent Self or to begin your practice of alternate nostril breath — as practiced in Week 1, Page 19.

3 – 5 minutes

Sink in. **Viparita Karani (Legs up the wall):**

Finish your practice with your legs up the wall or fully lying out on the floor — make it sweet.

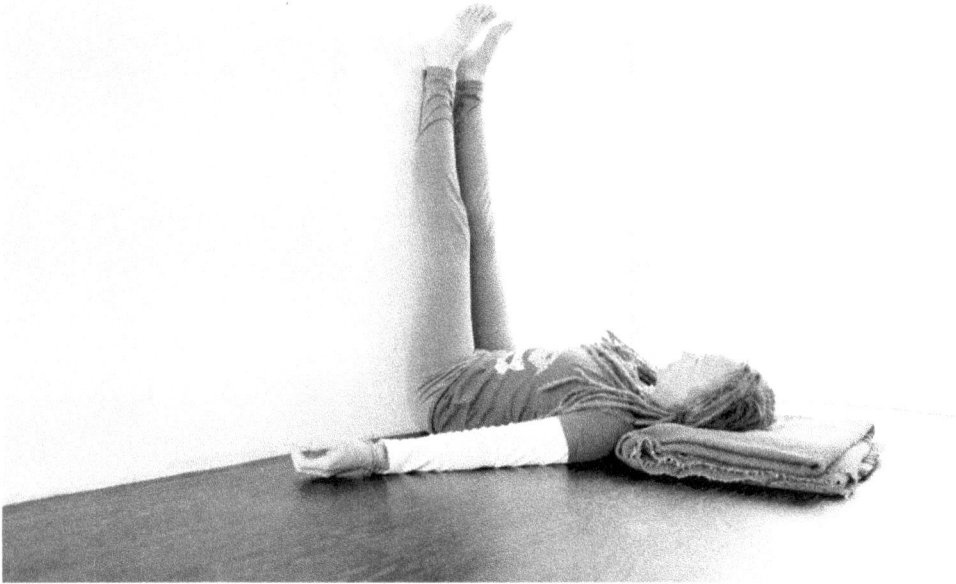

3 – 10 minutes (or until baby wakes)

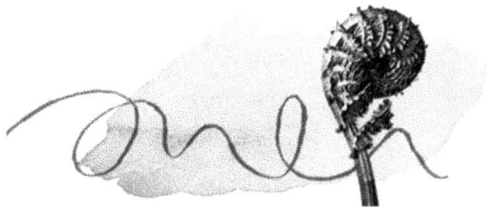

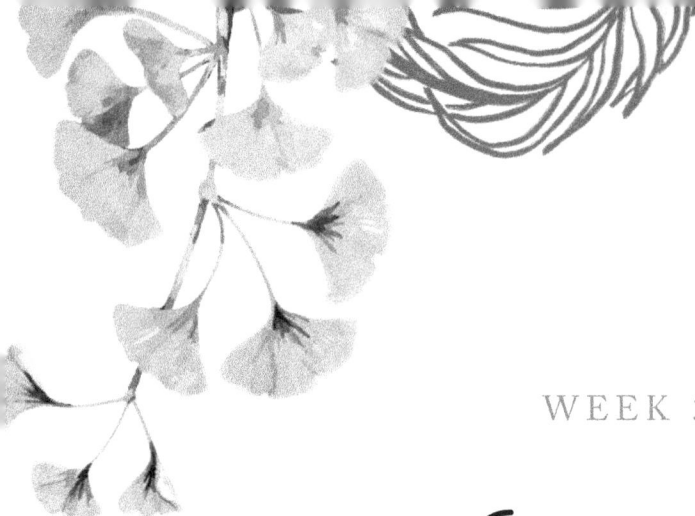

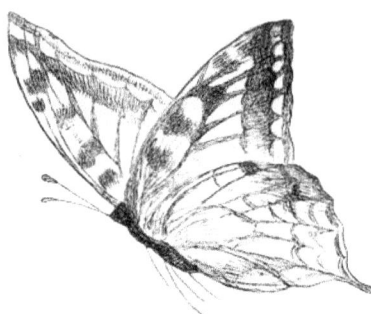

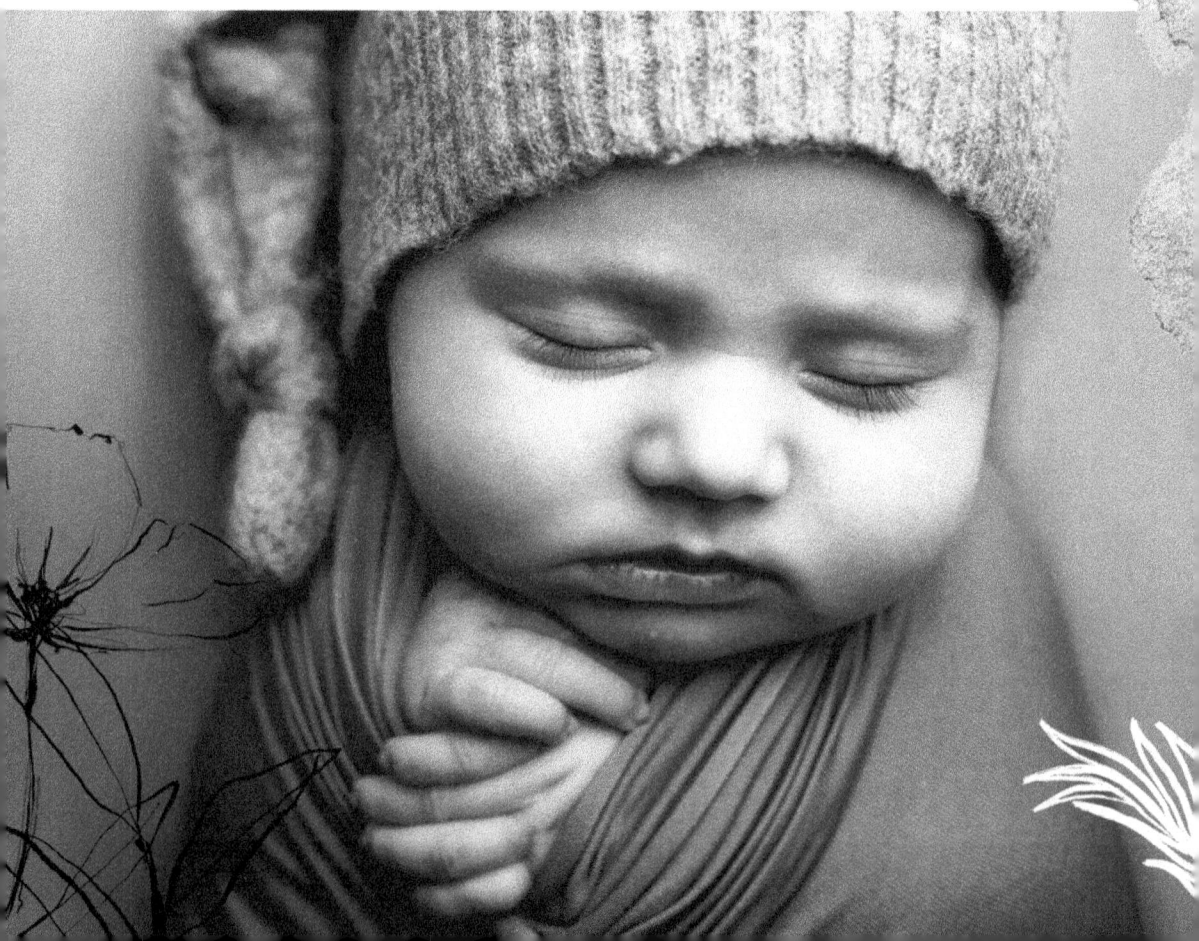

Emerging

*"Make your heart like a lake, with a calm still surface
and great depths of kindness"*

— Lao Tzu

Hard work and little sleep means your love and kindness must, first and foremost, be inwardly directed. The imminent return of your partner to work or perhaps the sad farewell to the freedom, spontaneity and boldness that previously defined you might move you to melancholy, fear, sadness, panic or anxiety. You might wonder just how you will get through the day... and the night. Overwhelmed, weepy, moody, intoxicated with love and deep gratitude, and all in the course of a single day. All of this, yet somehow, we muddle through... and eventually you will figure it out.

The seclusion patterns around the world in the weeks following birth keep a woman exempt from her usual world. They offer her nourishment and support as she turns in; to heal and become whole. Traditionally it was 30 days of chicken soup, tender care and the love and prayers of the village. In our current cultural fabric it can be reduced to just days, so deeply honour whatever time you do have. You may be barely brushing your teeth but you are doing the most important work of your life.

This third practice tempts you out just a little further, bringing you for the first time to your vertical Self and who you are now as you come to your full height, even if it's tentative, in these new days.

May your practice be the glue that binds you.
Breathe deeply daily. Seek kindness always

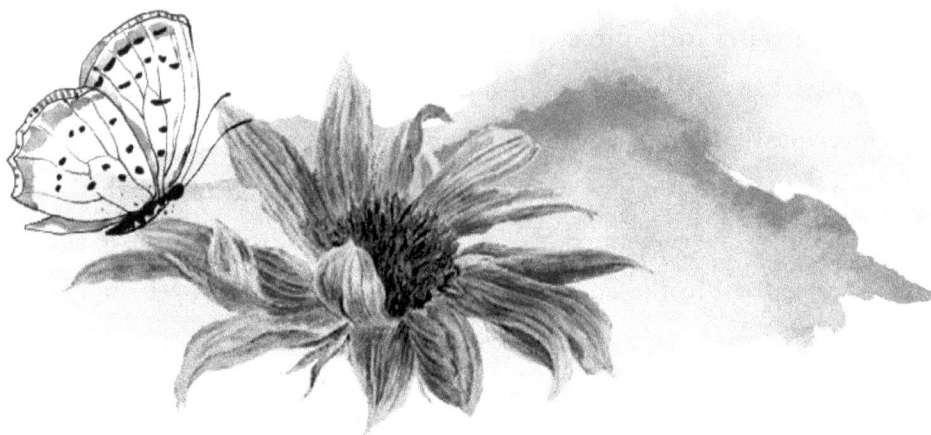

Coming home. **Child's pose variation:**

Start your practice in a childs pose observing your inner climate. The intensity of the emotional journey may be starting to fade and integrate into a better wholeness now. The bruising and battle scars of the body are healing sweetly, and here you are, a softer, more vulnerable version of yourself. It's an incongruent time where despite the deep shifts you have so recently experienced, trust is also beginning to grow in yourself, your circumstances and the natural mother you are becoming.

Find her and breathe life into her.

Child's pose gives us the perspective of the child: open, honest, inquisitive and gentle by nature. Embrace these softer qualities and allow them to draw you into the strength of what is light and playful within.

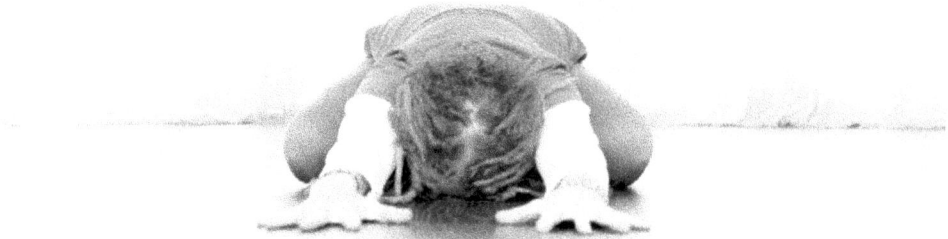

Come to child's pose with knees wide, big toes together, buttocks on the heels. Extend your chest forward along the floor. Arms reaching for the top of the mat or fold the back of the hands beneath your forehead.

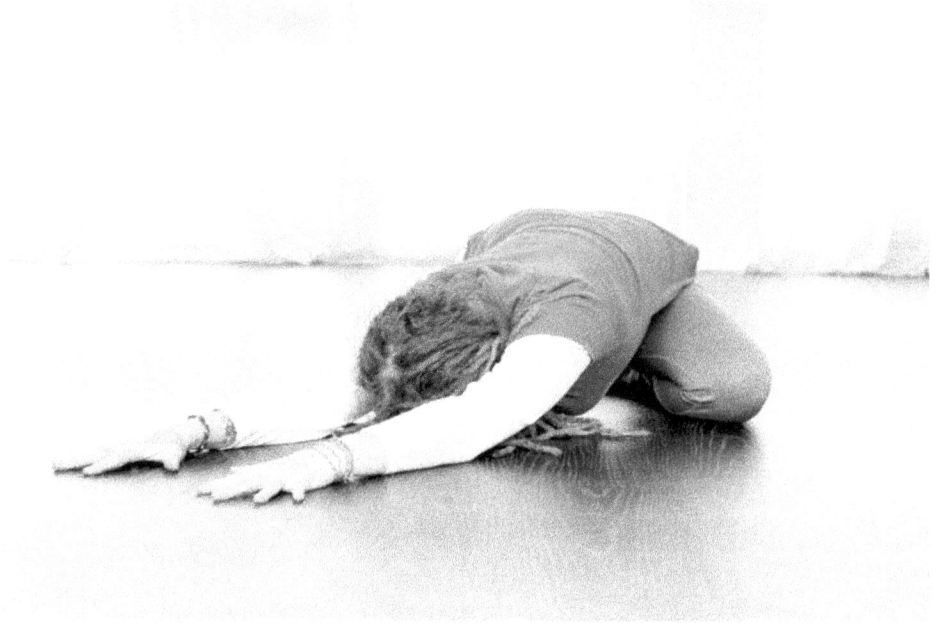

Exhale, walk the torso to the right. Take your breath into all the spaces in your edges. Pay particular attention to the spaces around the heart.

Hold for 3 – 5 breaths.

Inhale, and return to the centre.

Repeat on the opposite side.

Move from your centre. **Cat/cow variation:**

There's the physicality of moving into the sacred centre and then there's the energetics of it. Returning to centre can be something that mothers find elusive in the early weeks. Take your mind into the place you last left your centre, right under the navel, cast that influence, listen, and it will find you.

Move into all fours and into the cat/cow just as we did in week 2 only add a yoga block or rolled towel between your thigh bones. Squeeze a little — notice your lower back soothe.

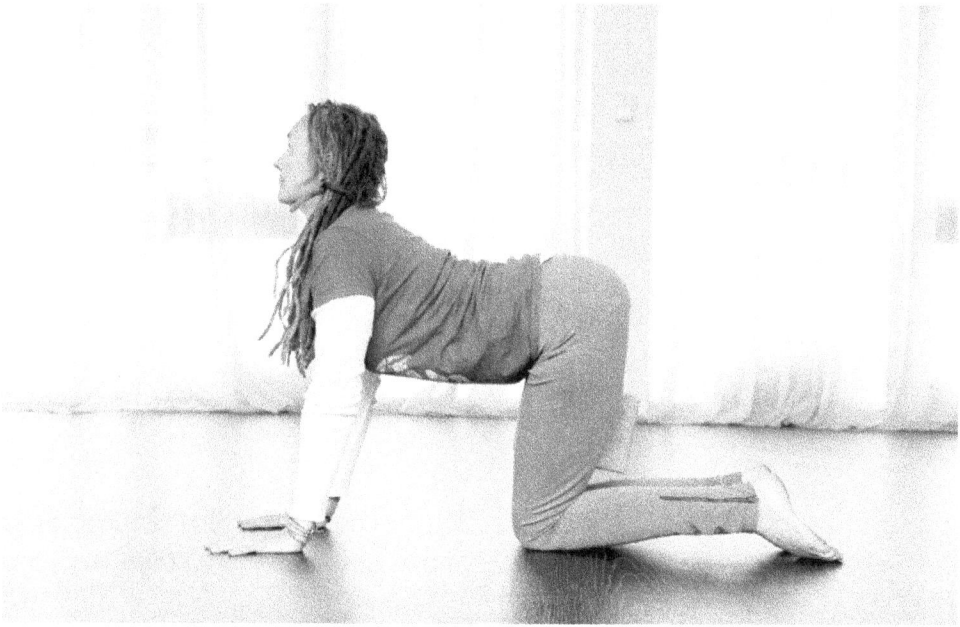

Inhale, look forward and open up the chest and feel the front body open as the tail lifts.

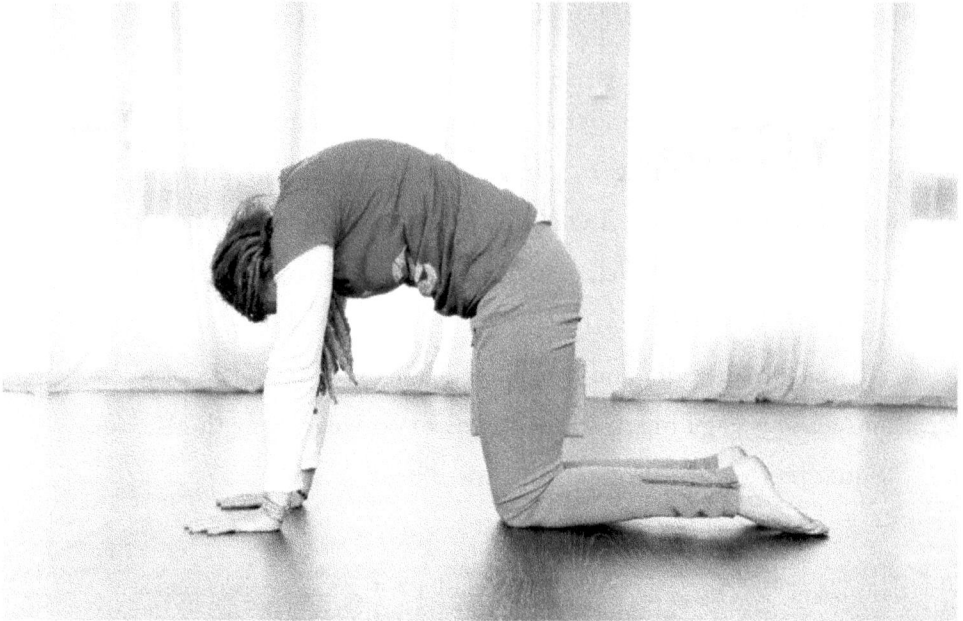

Exhale, arch the spine with chin tucked in, squeeze the block and feel the back spine open and the discs fill. As the breath empties and you apply pressure to the block, gently draw the navel in and upwards towards the spine. Imagine you are trying to make a hollow here.

Repeat 6 – 10 times with a smooth breath.

Return to child's pose to release. Remove the support from between the knees, wait for the rounding of the spine, hold the shape and inhale against it.

Exhale and roll the buttocks backwards, stretching the spine as you take them towards the heels. This time bend the elbows and rest the forehead on the back of the hands or fists and let the chest drop towards the floor. Stay here as long as you like, releasing the upper back and chest.

Coming from a strong place. **Spinal toning:**

With small but regular returns to the statesmanship of the back body, we continue to recalibrate our present in the light of the experience of our past. We mark out the constructs of the future from the place of wisdom and experience that exists behind us.

Return to your all-fours position.

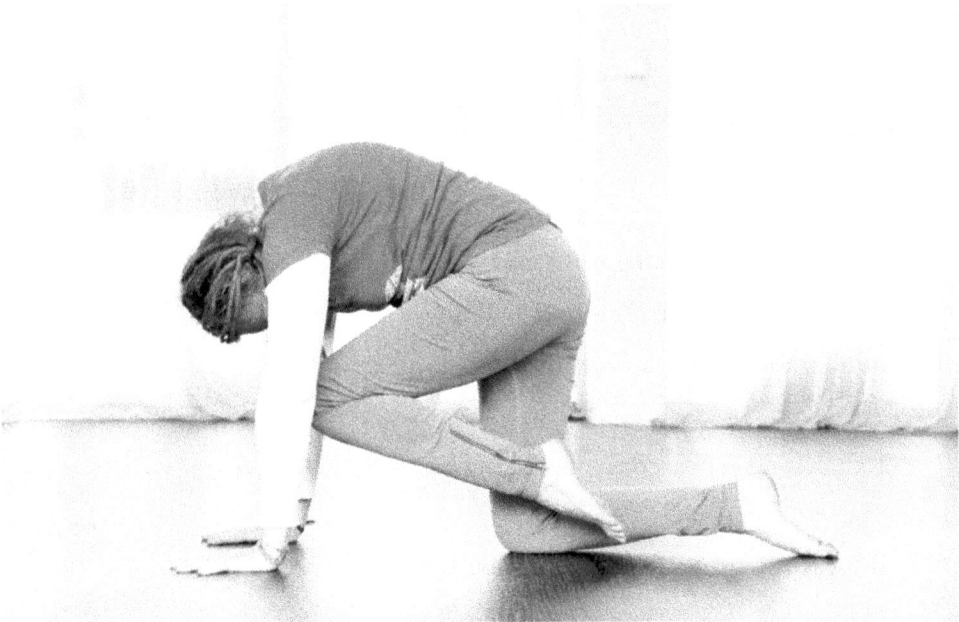

Exhale, cat arch the spine and draw the right knee in towards the forehead.

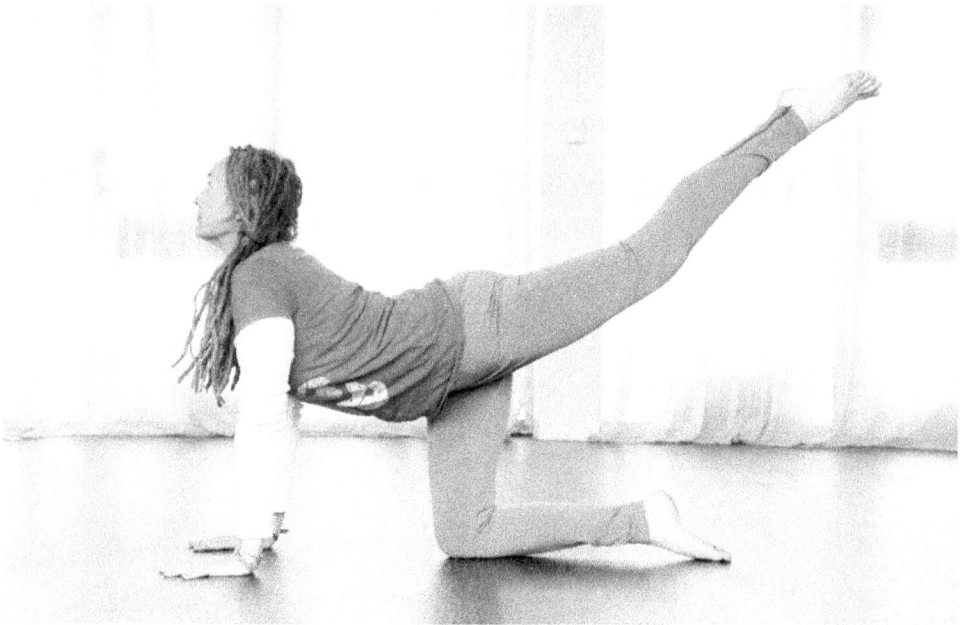

Inhale, and extend the right leg back, reaching it high and opening the back of the knee. Extend all the way into the foot. Feel the lumbar and buttock take up tone.

Exhale and repeat, drawing the knee to the forehead.

Repeat the cycle 4 – 8 times slowly with the breath.

Repeat on the opposite side.

If this feels too strong for you right now, repeat the alternating arm and leg position we did last week.

Take a rest in child's pose and allow the spine to provide a supporting neutral space into which the breath can settle.

Your moment of truth. **Adho mukha śvānāsana and variation (Downward-Facing Dog):**

This is the pose that most experienced yogis crave and most beginners dread. This is a soft or half version of the pose to be done with the utmost respect whether you are new to practice or not. At this point in the sequence its purpose is to relieve your upper back and give you a moment of celebration — of your strength, your commitment and of who you are becoming. Follow the out-breath for therein lies all the answers.

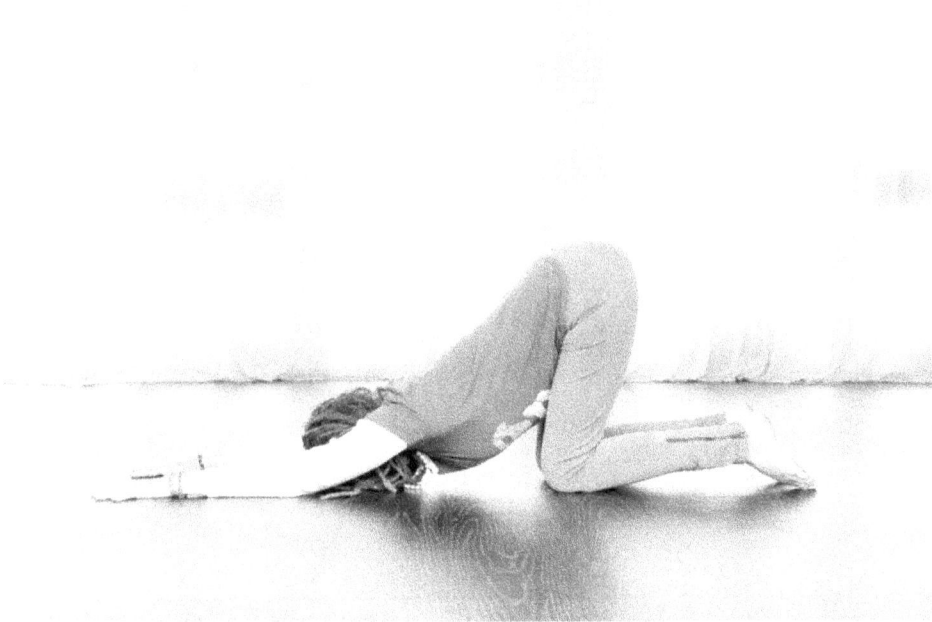

From all fours position walk your arms forward at shoulder width. Bend the arms at the elbows, sending them out to the left and right. Rest the forehead on the backs of the hands or extend the arms forward and feel the delight of the upper back spaces as they breathe. The buttocks may one day be over the knees, for now just be content with working them towards that space.

Hold here for 3 – 5 long breaths. Press back to child's pose briefly then return to all fours.

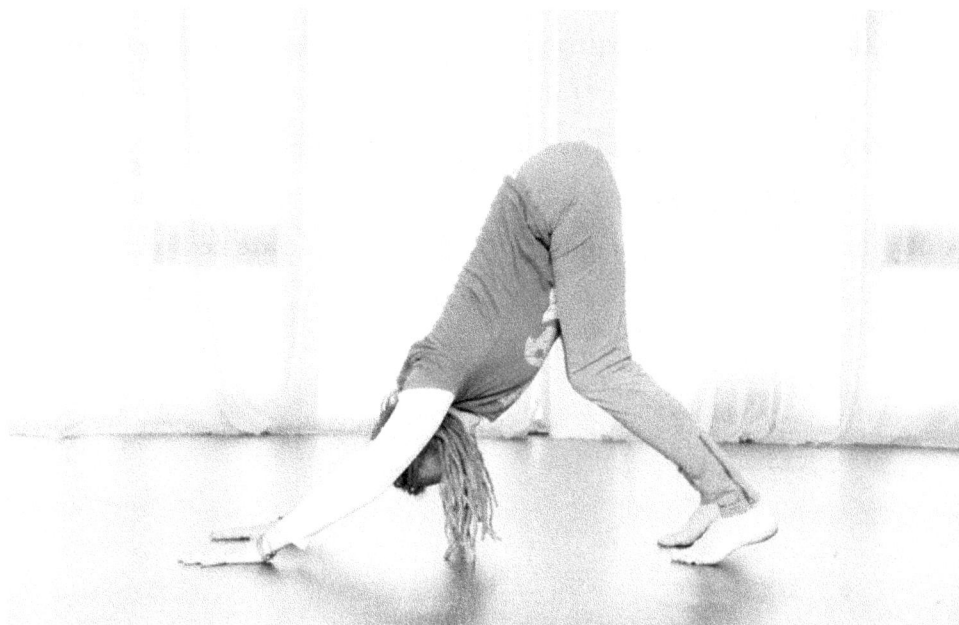

From all fours push up into a bent leg downward dog. Have your hands at shoulder width or wider, your feet in line with your hands, your knees 30 percent bent. Let your head hang as you press your arms down and forward into the floor to lengthen your spine.

Take 5 slow breaths here, opening the chest gently towards the thighs while keeping the arms active. Hold mindfulness in the alignment of the crown of your head and your tailbone to create a long spine. Attempt to lengthen the back of the legs softly one at a time with the breath, but only if if it doesn't hijack your spinal length.

If you aren't feeling the strength or alignment to be in this pose at this time repeat the first variation — the half dog.

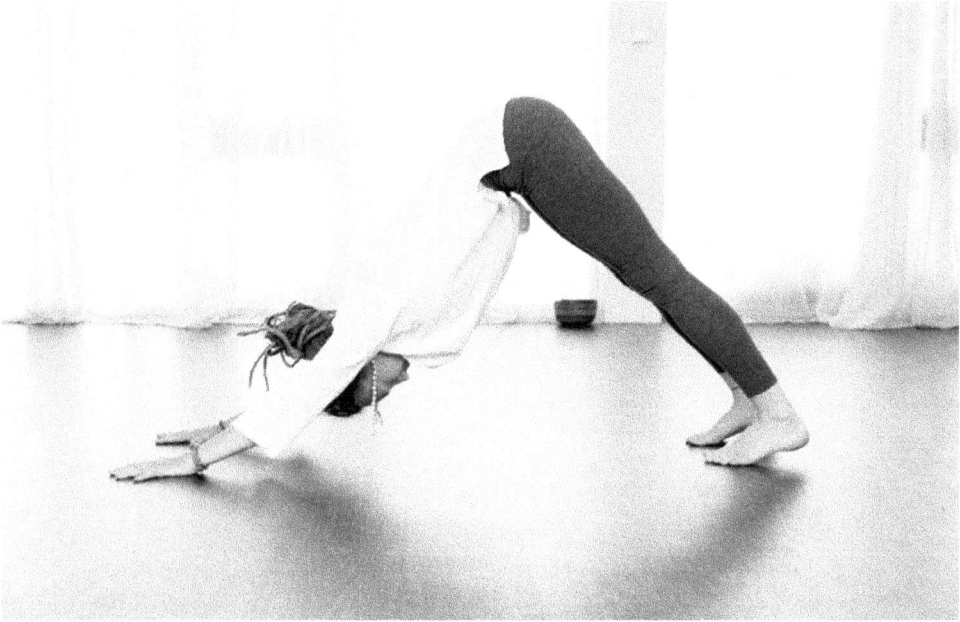

Straighten the legs and go all the way if it feels right for you.

Stay in this mild inversion for as long as it feels good and right, taking note of the belly as it breathes in and out at the navel centre.

Stepping into your luminescence.
Trikonasana (Triangle Pose):

This pose coaxes us out from the centre to feel for the edges of this new space you inhabit.

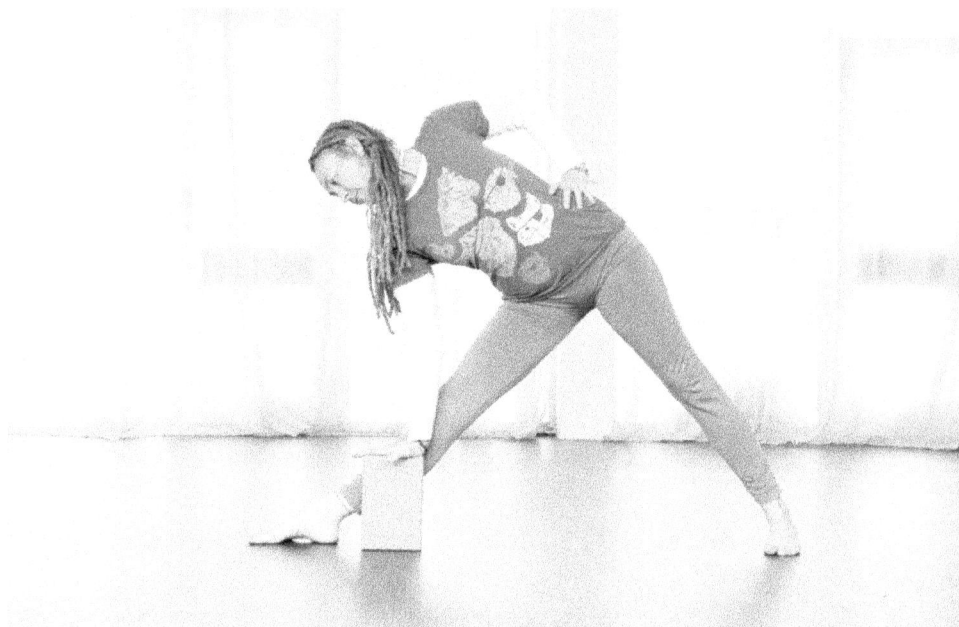

From downward-facing dog pose or all fours step your right foot forward between the hands. Turn the back foot at 45 degrees. Place the right hand at the right shinbone, yoga brick or knee. Left hand to your left hip.

Inhale, straighten* the front right knee, lengthen the spine and allow it to rotate the torso open to the left.

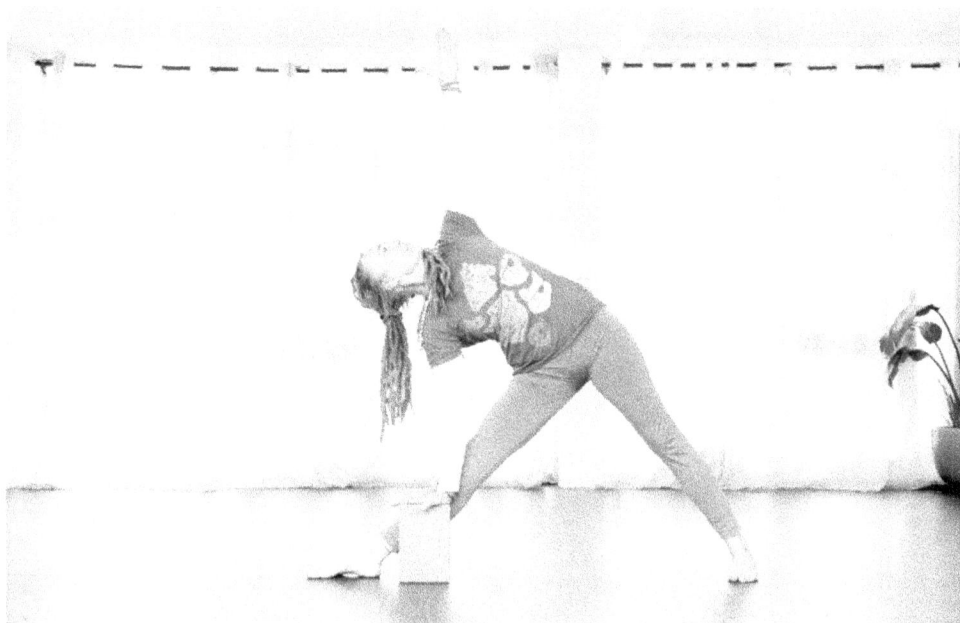

Exhale, and ground your sitting bones towards the backs of your knees to bed the pose down.

Inhale, rotate the torso around your centre to the left, and raise the top arm if comfortable.

Take 3 – 5 breaths here.

Step back to downward dog and repeat on the opposite side.

Straighten is the word here, without the leverage of the front leg the pelvis is turned down and compromises the spine and so the levity and lift of the whole shape. Use a yoga block, chair or other clever prop to raise the lower hand high enough from the floor for you to comfortably straighten the front leg. Micro bend the knee if you experience any pain in or around the joint.

Move in and under. **Uttanasana (Standing forward fold):**

After the edges comes the return. Uttanasana offers a place from which we can take rest and salvation. If it doesn't feel like salvation, bend your knees until it does.

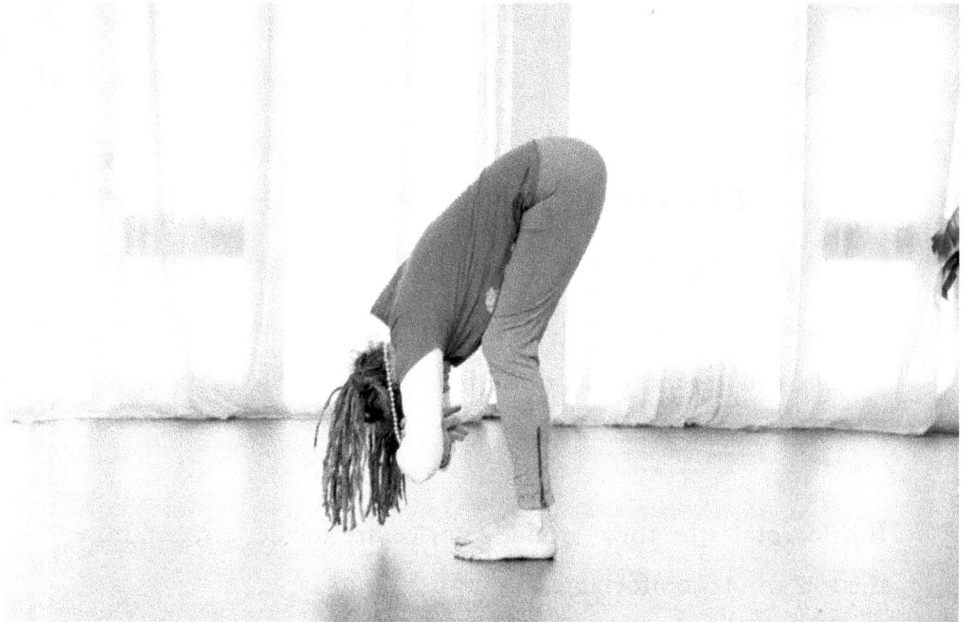

From downward dog, walk your hands backwards towards your feet. Have the feet at hip distance or slightly wider, and bend the knees to allow the torso to soften forward without strain, and the lower back to let go.

If your back body needs support keep your hands on the floor, however, you can extend the pose into the side ribs and upper back by interlocking the forearms as shown here.

If there is a wall behind you, drop the buttocks to the wall for support. Have the feet about 30 cm from the skirting board. Ensure the thighs and belly make contact for a gentle belly compression.

If you are tight in your back body, rest your hands on the nearest chair or sofa instead.

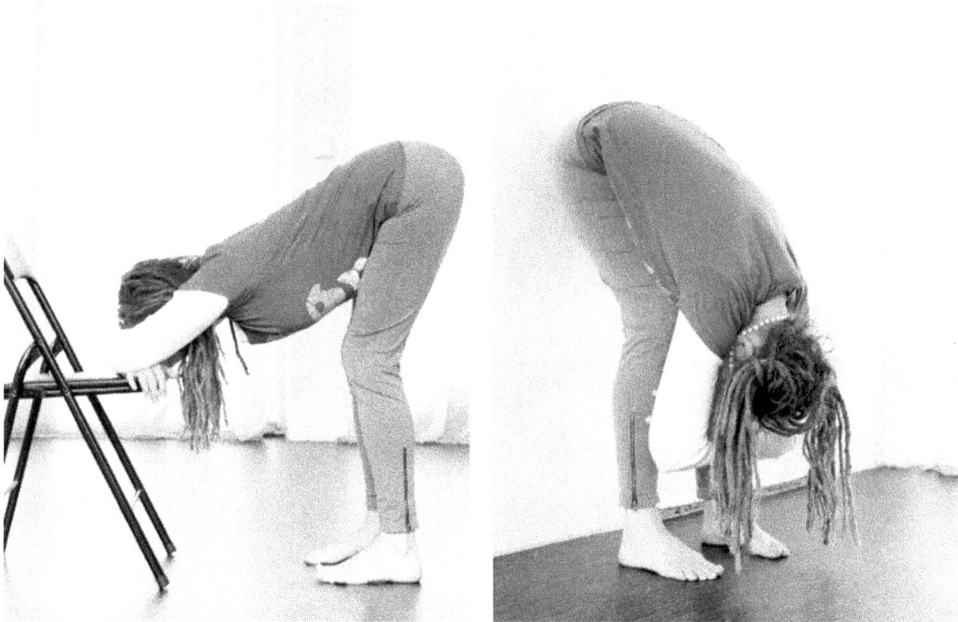

To make this pose even sweeter, place a rolled towel under the navel and fold forward over it offering compression for the belly and tone for the abdominal organs.

Take 5 – 10 breaths here before rolling up to stand at your full height, in all your power and grace.

* The wider the feet the greater the access to this shape. Feel free to experiment.

Reclaiming space. **Reclining twists:**

This twist series acts like a hydraulic pump through the dural fluids and disc spaces in the spine. In turn it allows the nervous system to float freely in its briny bath without interruption or impediment.

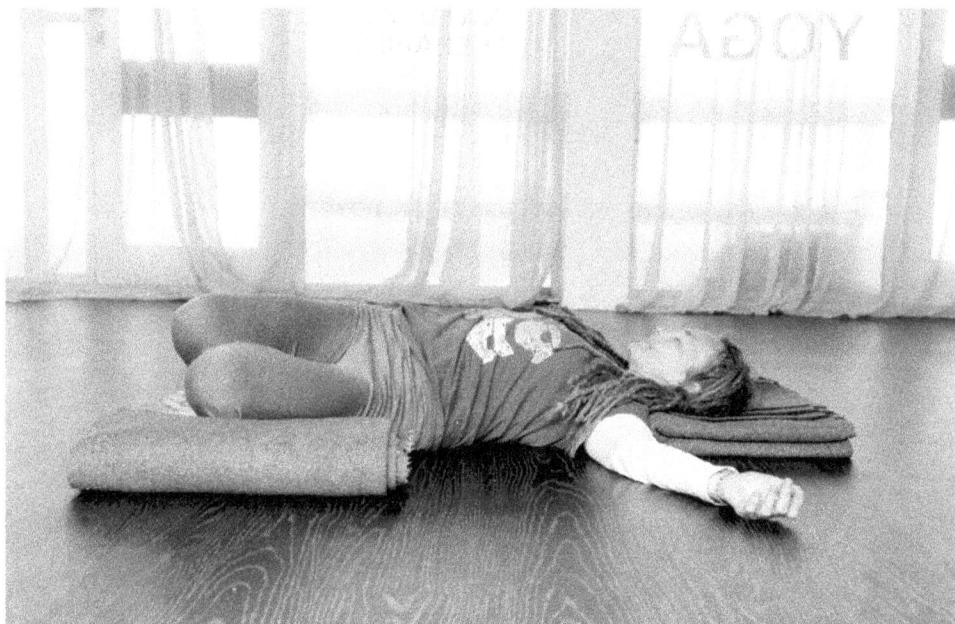

i) Lie on your back, knees bent, soles of the feet to the floor. Walk the inner lines of the legs together from ankles to inner thighs. Arms extend out at 90 degrees from your shoulders. To deepen, bring your arms into a cactus position with elbows at a 90 degree bend, either way ensure both shoulder blades are on the floor.

Exhale, and drop the knees to the right. Keep your shoulder blades down so you can release the spine from top to bottom. Inhale and centre.

Repeat from side to side 6 – 8 times.

To deepen the work of this pose after a few repetitions hold the knees over to the right. Place a rolled blanket under the outer knee to give a little lift and support. Look to the left if the neck is comfortable.

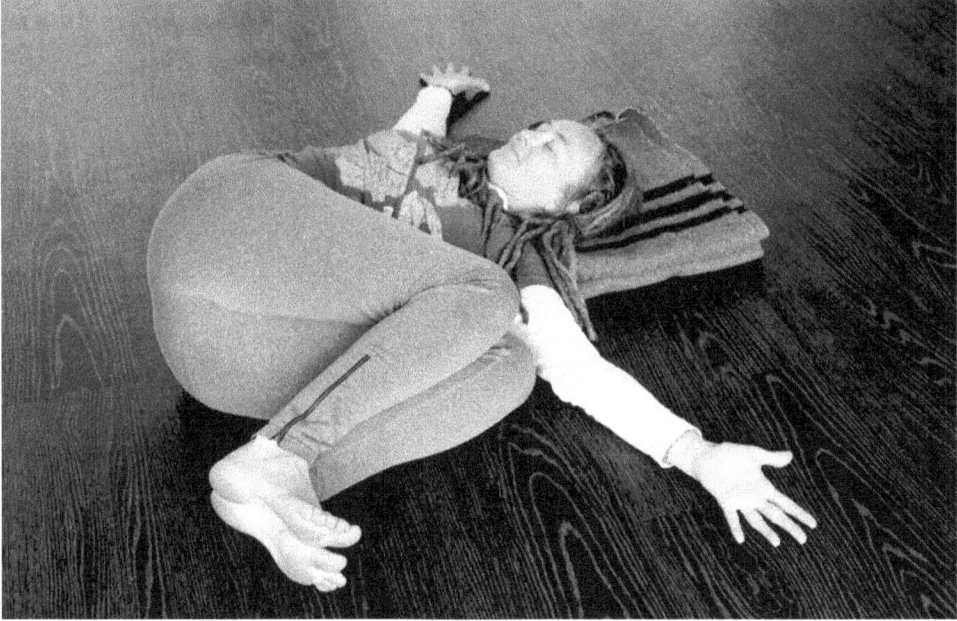

Hold this shape allowing the body to fall into its container for 1 minute.

Repeat on the opposite side.

ii) From the same supine position draw the knees up to the chest and repeat as above, aiming the knees as high as you can towards the armpits. This will give you a deep and thorough upper back release.

Rest lying on your back for a few breaths after this sequence is complete. Allow it time to integrate.

Now—let it go. **Supported setu Bandha (Bridge Pose):**

You may decide this pose is your favourite, offering up a balance for the folding down that happens when learning how to breastfeed and soothe. It lights up your inner spaces, expands your breath and invites us into an attitude of great grace.

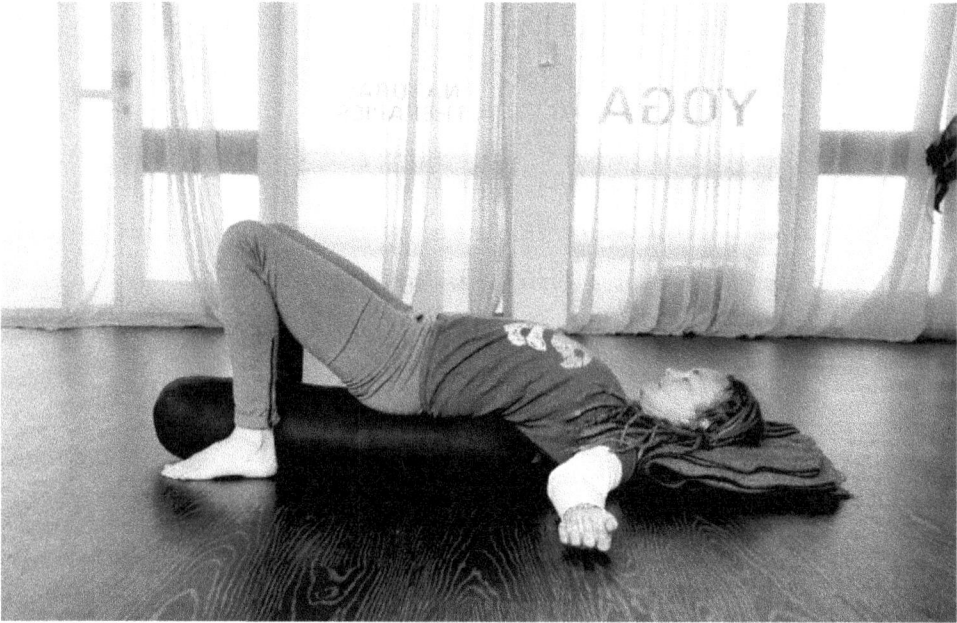

Use a folded blanket or bolster to raise the spine, support the head on a second blanket if necessary. With your buttocks just forward of the bolster's edge, lay yourself over its length. Head and shoulder blades are on the floor. Gently tuck your shoulder blades under and down and extend your arms out to the sides at shoulder height. You may like to leave your legs out long, be in an easy-cross position or feet on the floor with knees to the ceiling. It should feel good.

You can deepen the pose by taking the arms overhead and gently holding your opposite elbows.

Stay here for 1 – 3 minutes

To exit the pose, roll to the side and off your supports. Return to lying on your back and hug your knees to your chest, rocking gently side to side to disperse.

This pose should feel amazing. If it's uncomfortable in your lower back, try wriggling down off the prop a little. If it's uncomfortable in the neck or upper back, place a higher support under the head. If it feels like it's too strong across the chest, lower the back support so you have less height to span.

Return to the centre. **Cross leg forward fold:**

As the weeks go by this return becomes easier and easier. It invites you to stay and hang out for a while, it calls your deepest yearnings to the surface where you can see them and, when the time is right, make them manifest.

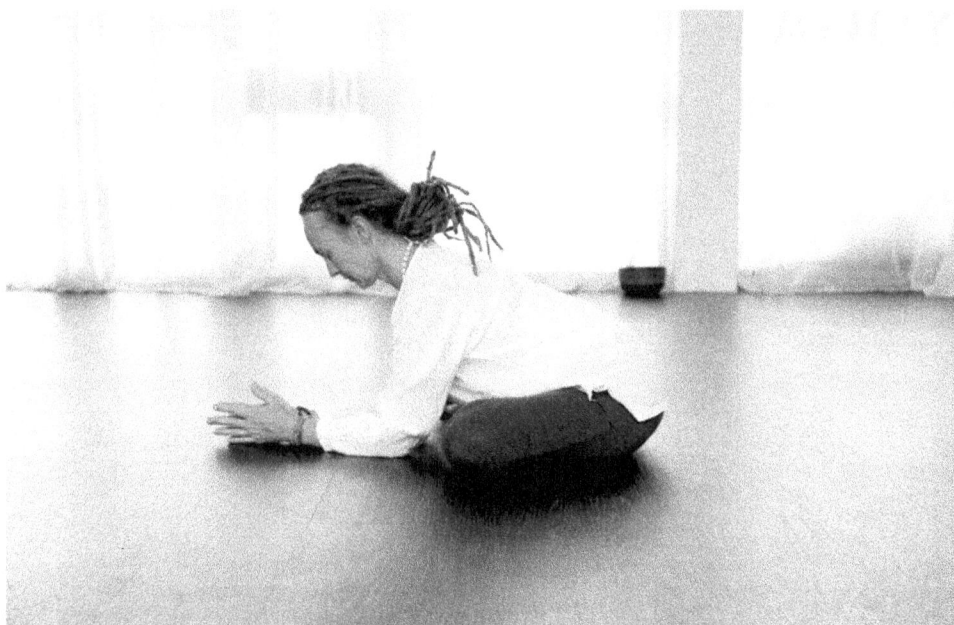

Raise the torso and come to a seated easy cross-leg position or sit in a chair. Raise the buttocks on a cushion if necessary. Exhale, and allow the torso to come forward towards the floor in front of you.

Inhale, lengthen and align the spine from crown to tail.

Exhale and soften the forehead onto a chair, yoga block, cushions or floor.

Hold for 1 – 3 minutes. Change the cross of the legs and repeat on the opposite side.

Deep rest. **Savasana:**

Either have your legs up the wall or lie on your back. Allow
the body/mind to drift with the breath. Feel the lightness and
silence generated by your practice and be rewarded with a sense
of restoration and repair.

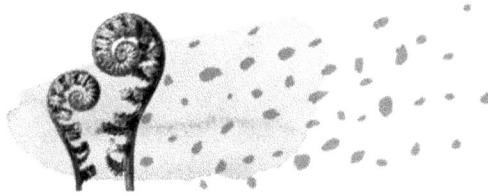

The Mother Lion

"It's come at last," she thought, "the time when you can no longer stand between your children and heartache."
—Betty Smith, *A Tree Grows in Brooklyn*

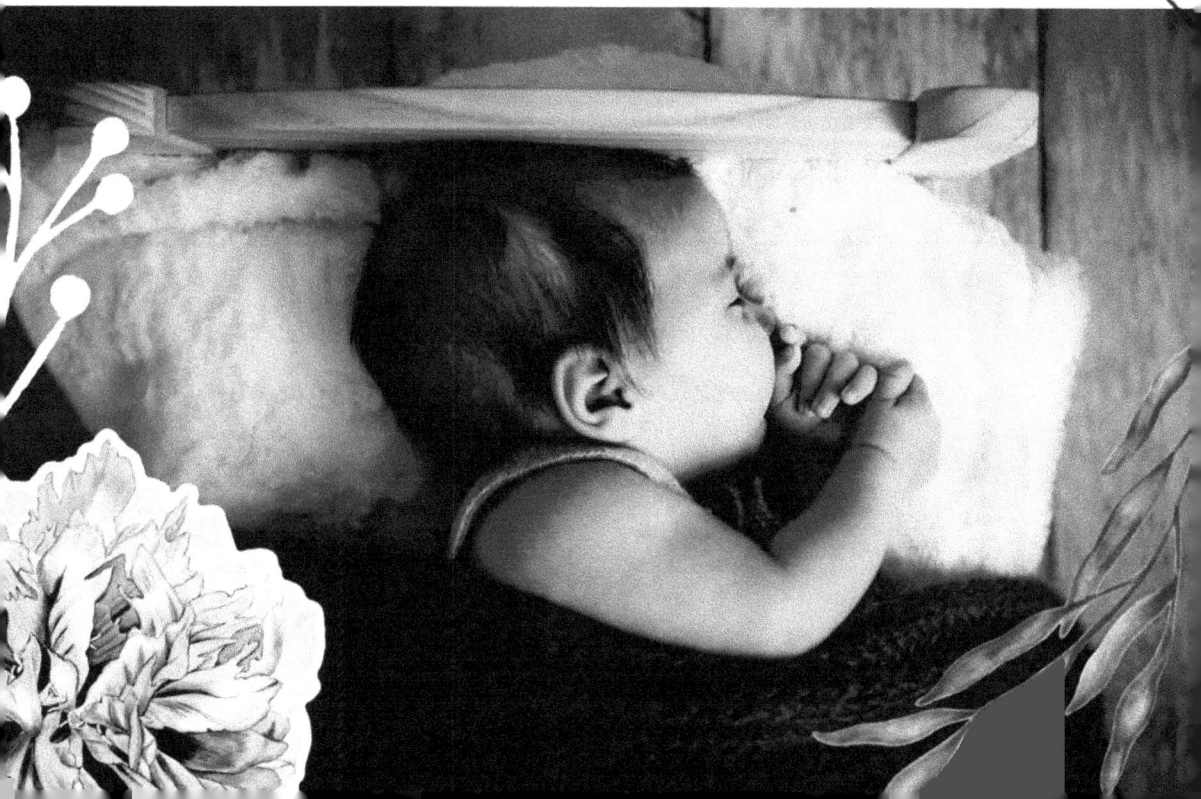

Discovering motherhood is a circular and successive process. A life transition that embodies expansion and contraction, destruction and integration, disorganisation and reorganisation. As each of these experiences are slowly assimilated, they become the foundation of the new 'Mother' self.

At each turn it seems everything we thought we knew becomes open to change. Some changes will cross over neatly, others will become crystallised, and others will dissolve completely. This allows us into the dance of transition and fluid change that is growth and personal development.

You, Dear Heart, are being pushed onto the path least trodden. Motherhood calls you to take your wheel out of the rut that is known and familiar and courageously take another path. We can try to grasp the pieces of the world we once knew but it has been replaced with another current, one that urges you out of your wild mind and invites you to see the fertile ground you are standing on. The beauty in this unfamiliar place.

At times it may feel like we are sitting in the rubble of our old lives, forgetting for a moment that we wished for this. It's ok to have these thoughts, they are the sandpaper that works away at our rough edges. These thoughts and feelings come to remind us that we are shifting and growing in powerful ways. It helps to remember and honour the divine being that you are and to have trust that all you have called forward is perfect. These early days are your realignment, have faith that you are exactly where you need to be. Go slow, sit under a tree, give yourself the time and space needed. All really is well.

Embrace this brave Lioness for she is a rare and beautiful creature, and go about this life's work with a sense of honour and pride for you are magnificent indeed.

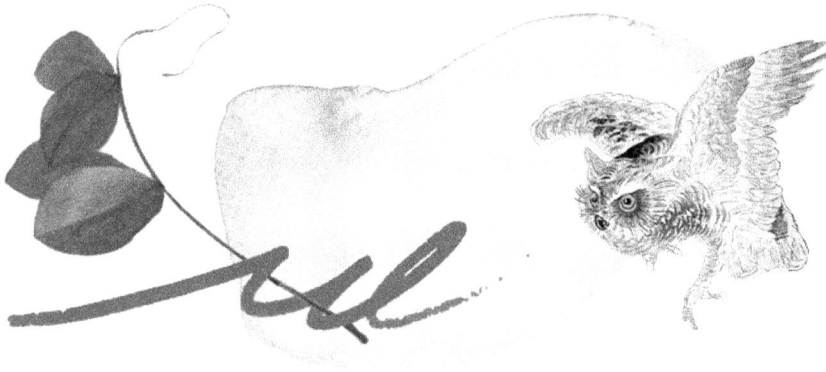

Start at its edges. **Side bending variations:**

Practice is always a winding in of sorts. Begin at the beginning, and end up somewhere completely different. In this spirit, starting at the edges of the container of the body is a simple metaphor for starting wherever you are today.

Come to a comfortable easy cross leg position. Find your base by reaching through the sit bones into the floor and follow the wave upwards to your crown. Notice that you are finding yourself more and more.

Extend the fingers out to the sides of the body, brushing your fingertips to the mat.

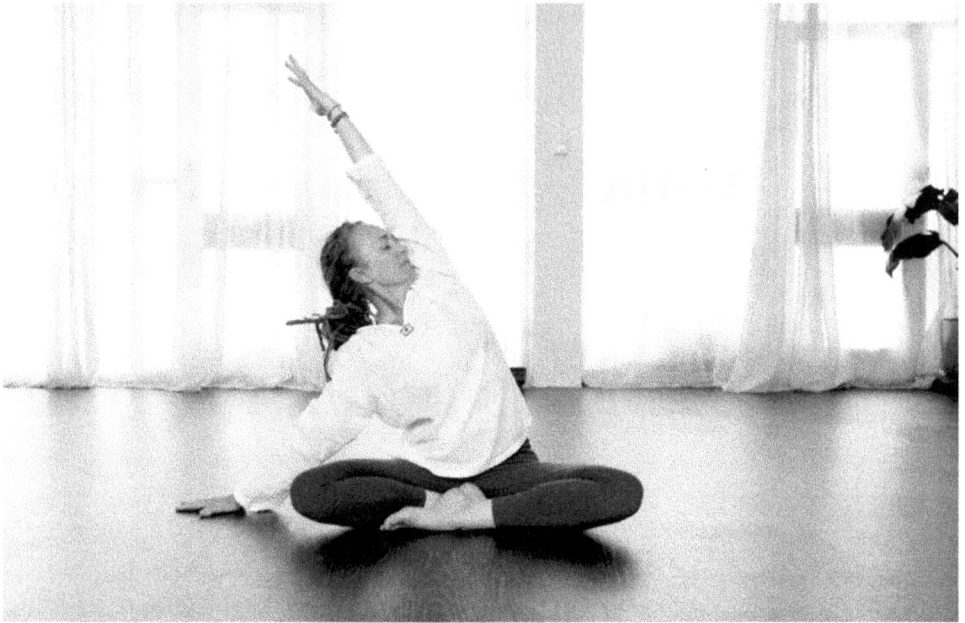

Exhale, place the right palm on the mat and raise the left arm up and over in a side bend to the right.
Inhale and return to centre.

Exhale and repeat on the opposite side.

It is intelligent practice to occupy the felt sense in lateral unwinding. Your body reveals its holdings and its sighs as you move through the occupied spaces. Slow down, deepen your breath and embody whatever rises with each passing.

Continue like this moving rhythmically from side to side for 8 – 10 breaths before returning to your still centre.

Gather and descend.

Sukhasana & Gomukhasana (Seated forward folds):

Gravity draws all things towards it; we are no different. By following that pull downwards we can more easily find our ground. By ground I mean steadiness, ease and familiarity in wild and changing times.

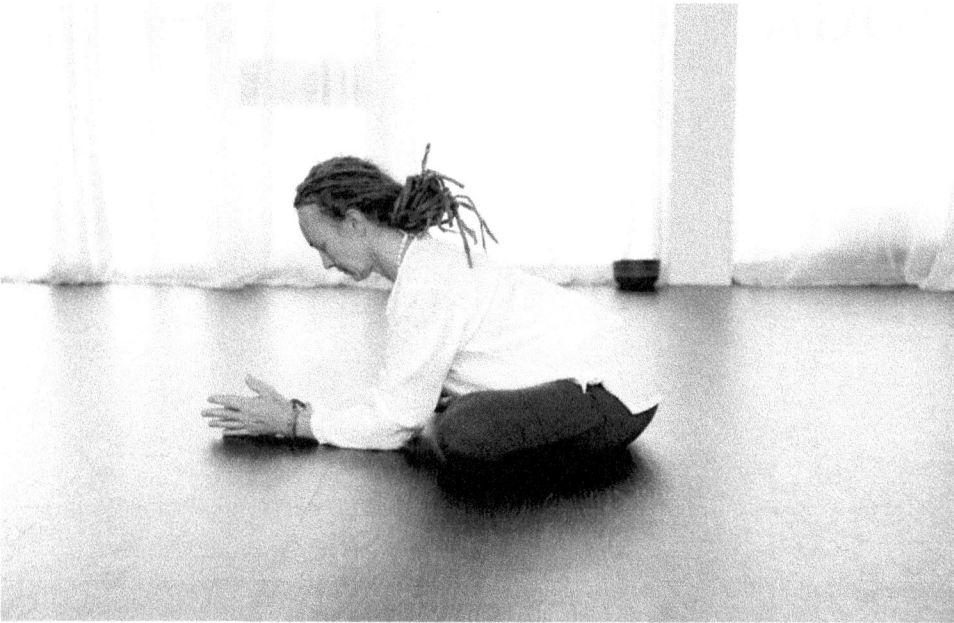

i) Remaining in the easy cross position from the previous pose, extend and open the chest forward as you attentively drop the torso a little way towards the floor. Your hips and lower back will be the barometer of your depth. Support the weight of the body on your hands or forearms. Take the pose to where the release in the sacral and outer hip area feels pleasant and nourishing.

Growing and birthing a child brings us face to face with the deepest and most hidden parts of our bodies, our sacral currents and the experiences from our mothers' wombs and our own primary cell division. When we offer breath and presence into these spaces we clear and bring light as we go. In this way we are opening ourselves to the pathway of reconciling all that has gone before, and healing all that is yet to come.

Hold for 8 – 10 breaths. Change the cross of the legs and repeat on the opposite side.

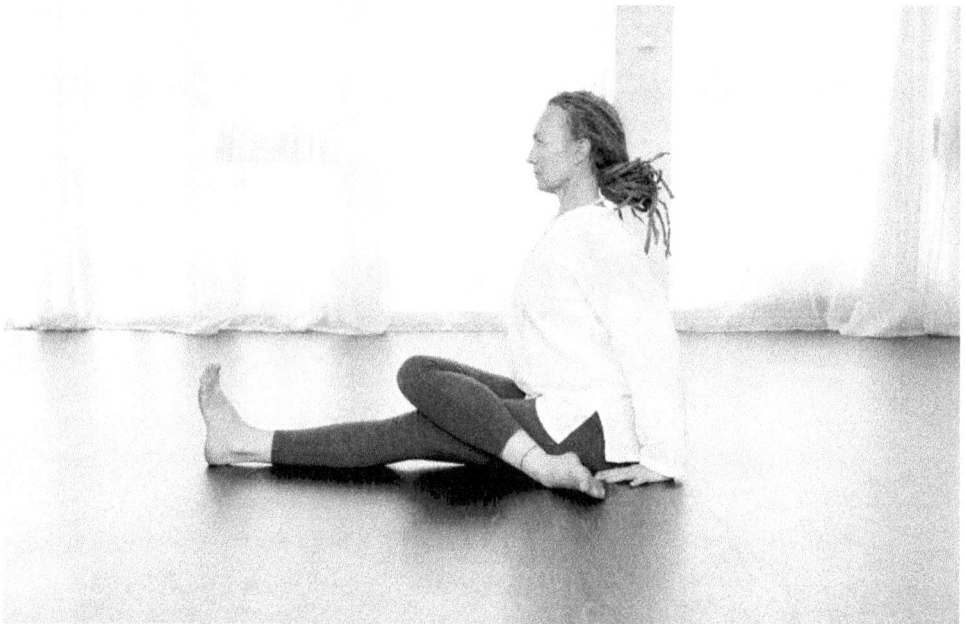

ii) Deepen the work by extending the legs forwards and out long, then folding the right leg so the right foot comes to the outer left hip with the knee facing straight ahead. Stay like this, or to deepen, fold the left leg underneath the right, bringing the left foot to the outer right hip. It provides a deep internal rotation of the hips.

Exhale twist to the right.

Inhale, and lengthen your spine inside the twist from the ground up. Hold for a few breaths.

Exhale (sigh), and return to centre.

Slowly drop forward through the layers of the hips.

Take 10 breaths to find your comfortable limit.

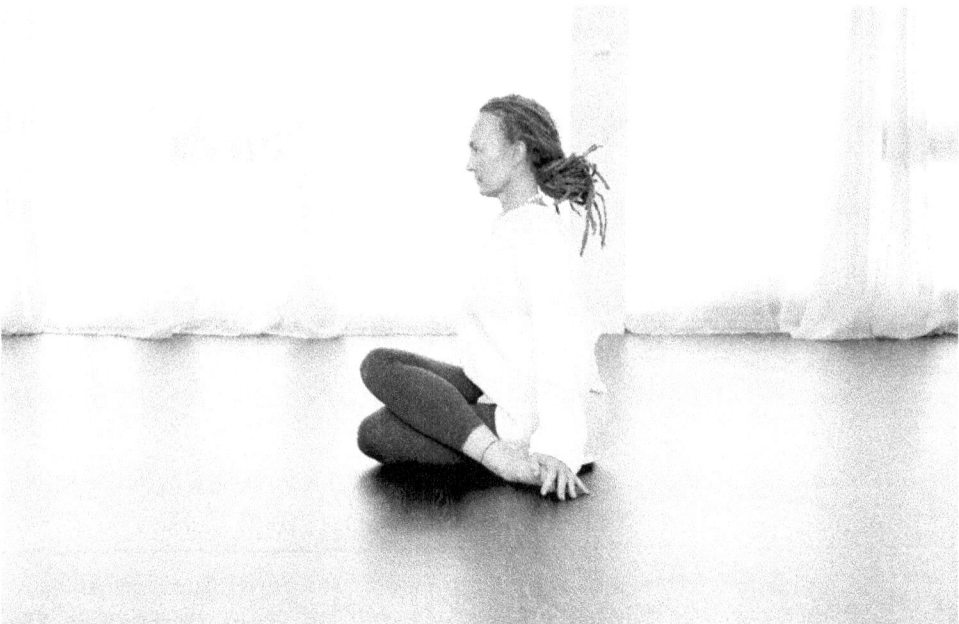

Repeat on the opposite side.

Unfold yourself to downward-facing dog pose to allow the warmth of blood to flow downwards into the legs.

Horizons.

Parivritta Parsvokanasana (High lunge with twist):

All standing poses offer up the alchemy of turning our Earth to the Sky. The more you find the yield into gravity, the greater the height, brightness and levity you can attain. By staying tethered and grounded in your base, you reach your full height.

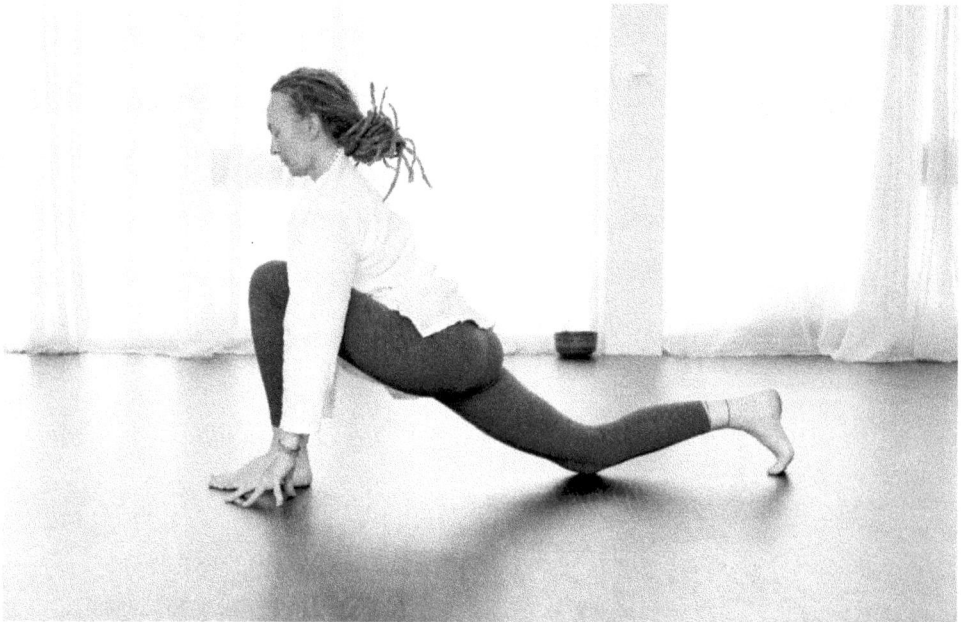

From downward-facing dog, step the right foot forward between the hands, choose whether to drop your back knee to the floor in a bent-leg lunge (as above) or keep the knee lifted in a straight-leg variation. Be guided by your strength and flexibility today. Keep both your hands on the mat.

Take 3 – 5 breaths here, trying to draw the pubic bone gently up towards the navel and the lower ribs in. Feel how the crown moves away from the sacrum and the front body supports the back.

Leave the left hand on the floor under the shoulder or place it on a block or other lift. Place the right hand on the right knee. Turn the upper body to the right while at the same time grounding the hips and legs downward. Raise the top hand to the roof if you feel the space. The focus should be in the upper back, chest and shoulders.

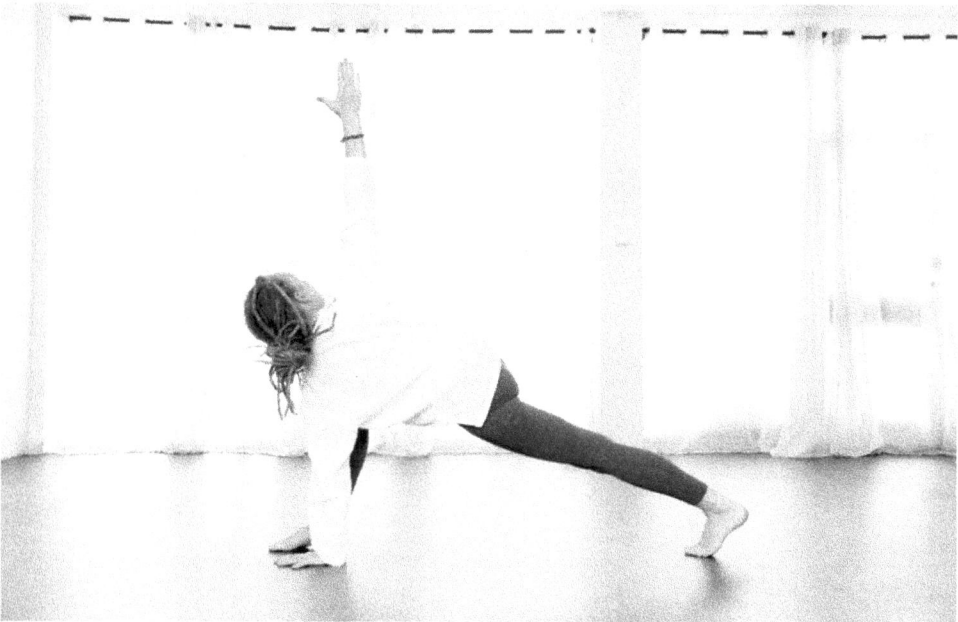

Take 3 – 5 breaths here.

Return to the straight or bent-leg lunge, then step back to downward-facing dog or all fours. Repeat with the left foot forward.

Rest: Depending on your energy levels either step the feet to the front of the mat and come to a soft-knee forward fold or drop the knees to the floor and rest in child's pose.

Warm the joints, steady the mind.
Simple salutation practice:

It's actually a salutation to the breath not so much the body so allow that to be your focus as the body just follows along. Continuing until the thoughts drop away, we wrap the movement of the body around the rhythm of the inhale and exhale. Here there is no effort and all is viscous flow.

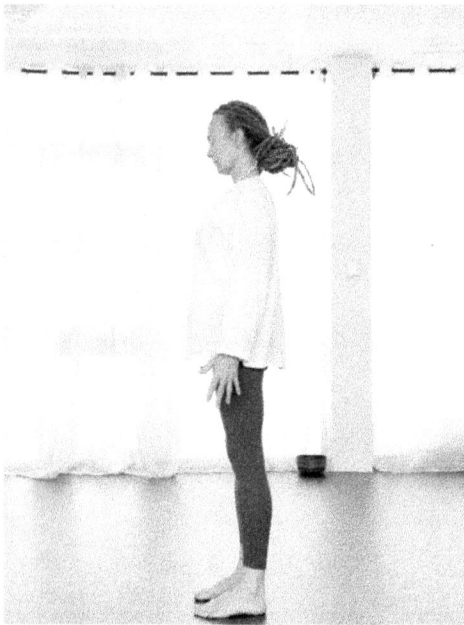

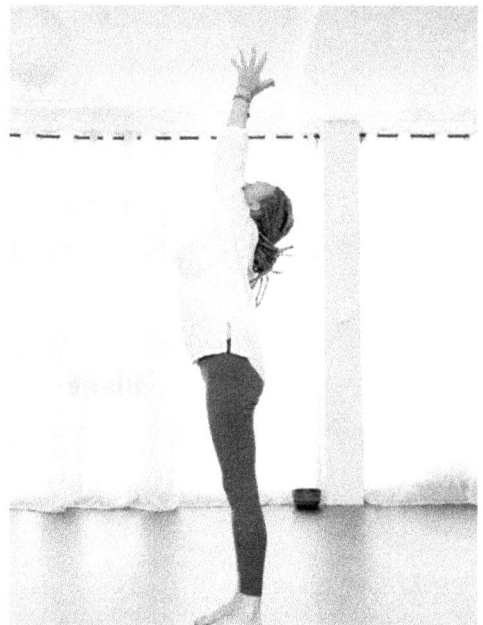

Come to a standing position at the front of the mat, feet together, hands by your sides. Be the Mountain.

Inhale and raise the arms up overhead, palms together if you can.

Exhale and fold into a standing forward bend, hands to the floor (bend the knees until the belly and the thighs touch and feel the press back of one against the other).

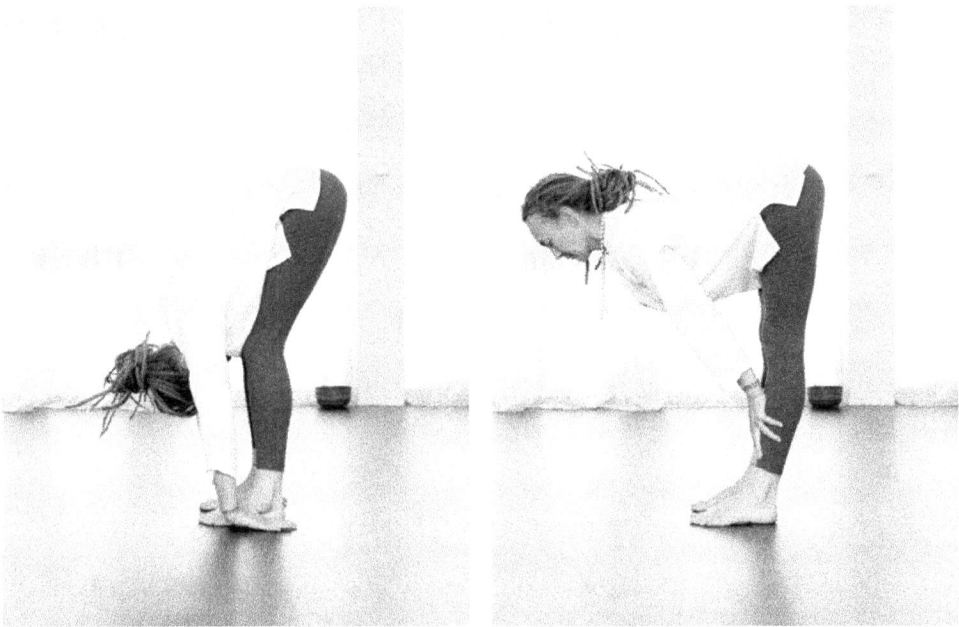

Inhale and ground the hands to the fronts of the shins, look forward and lengthen the spine. Attempt to straighten the legs here if it feels good.

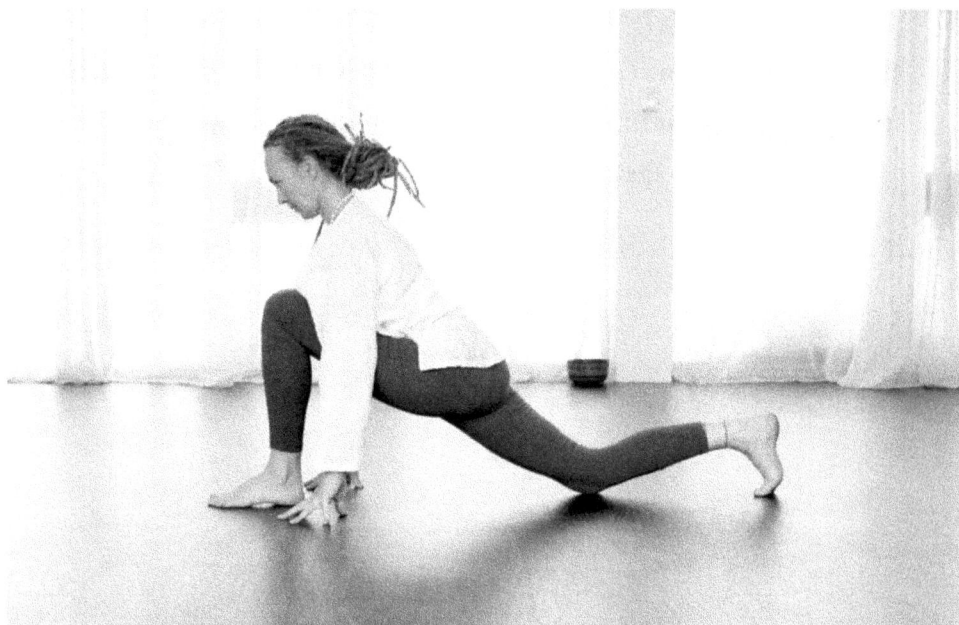

Exhale and step the right leg back to the end of the mat into the same lunge position we used earlier. It can be high or low — your choice.

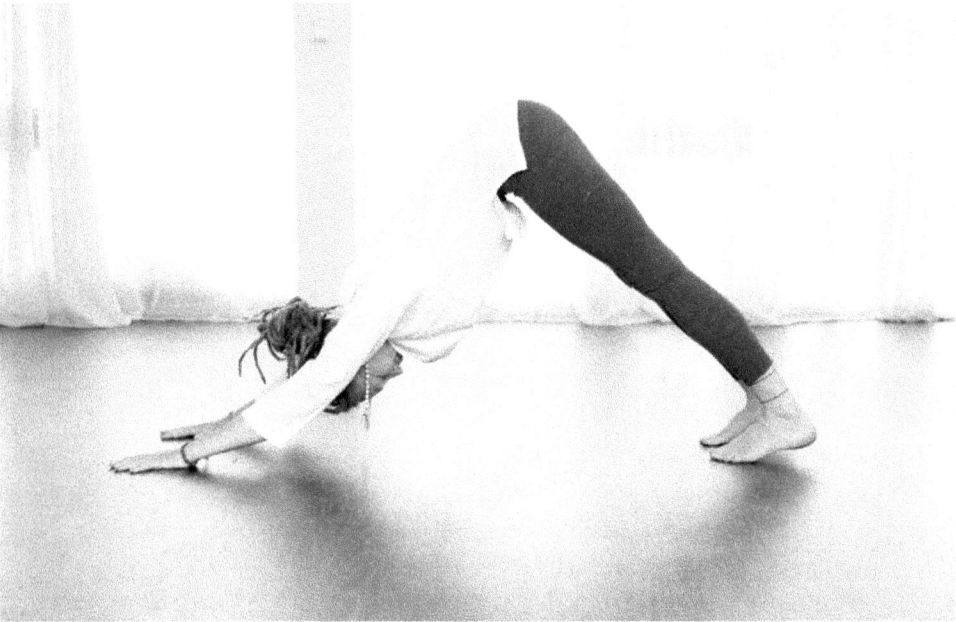

Inhale step to downward-facing dog by taking the left leg back to meet the right.

Hold here. Exhale, press your hands forward and your sitting bones back and find your space in the centre of the salutation. You may choose to stay here and take 5 breaths. You may even choose a child's pose here.

Now we go back the way we came.

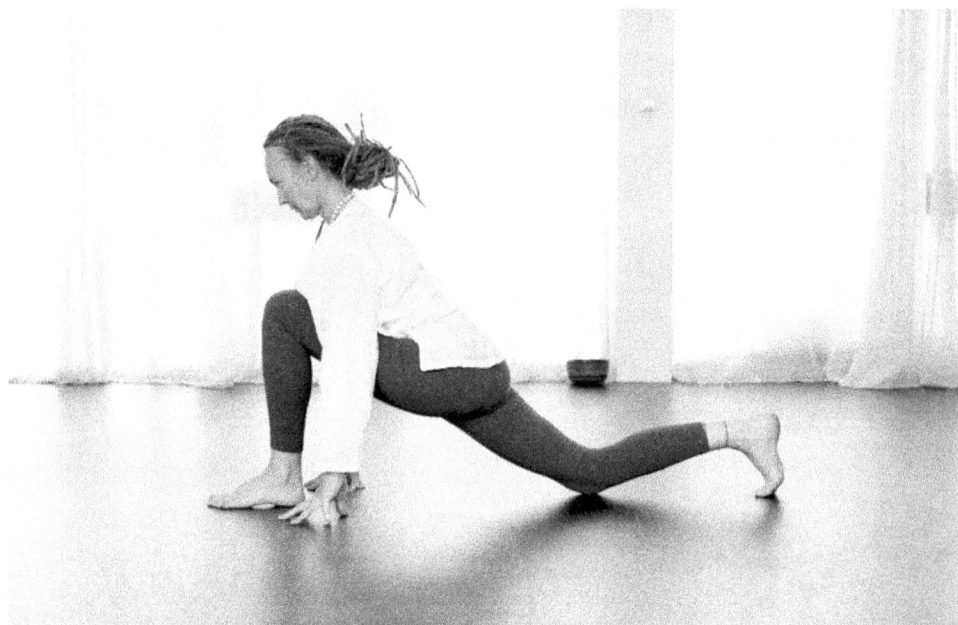

Exhale, step the right foot between the hands into a lunge position.

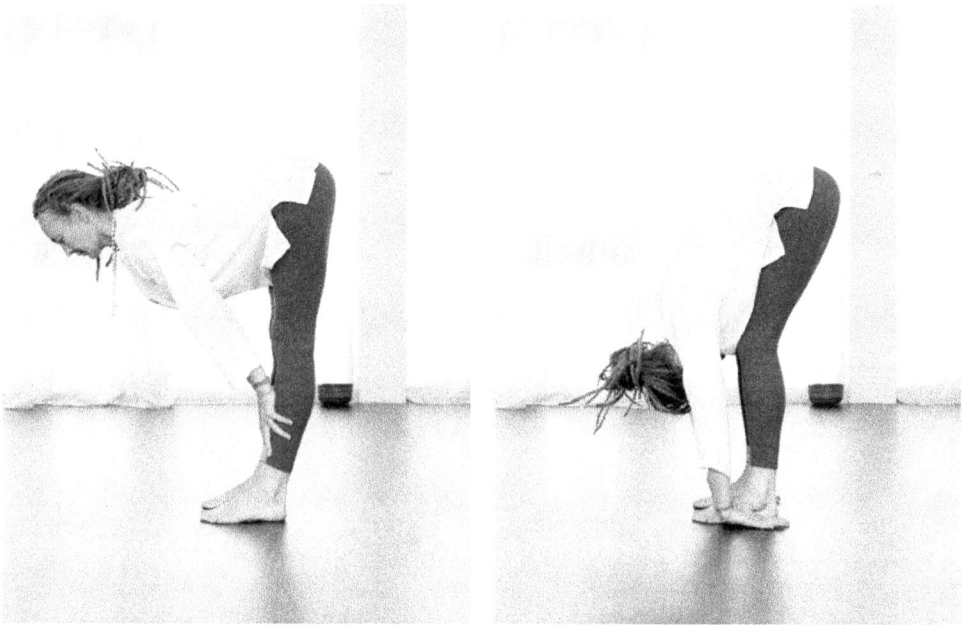

Inhale, step the left leg forward and look upwards with your hands on your shins or the floor like a half forward fold. Feel the upper back and chest release.

Exhale, and soften forward into the forward bend. Feel the belly gently compress against the thighs as you lift the navel back towards the spine just a little.

Inhale and breathe into your sides

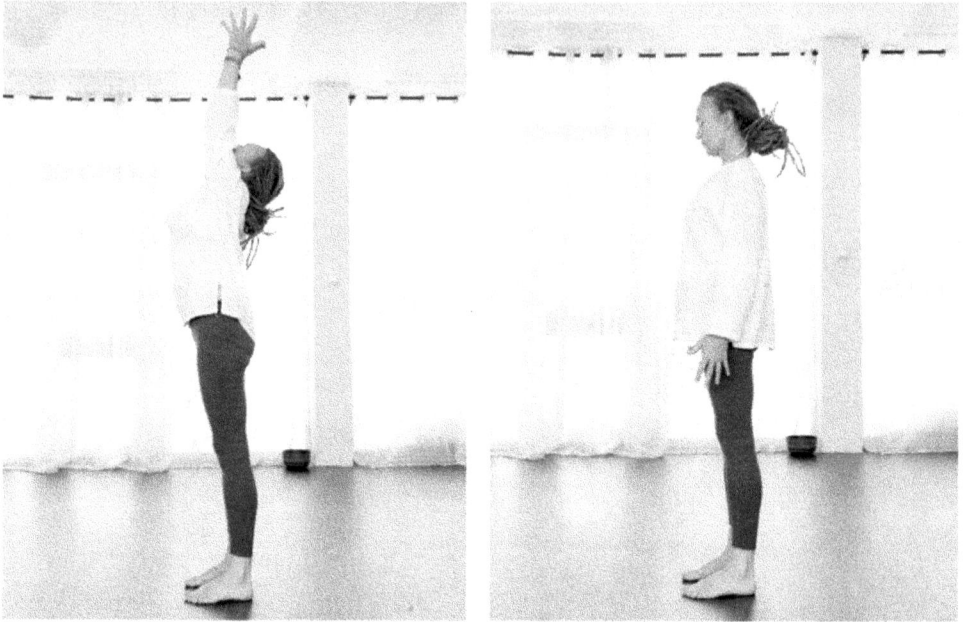

Exhale and slowly roll to standing with the chin drawn in and knees bent.

Inhale, raise the arms and create a soft standing backbend.

Exhale andreturn to standing.

Repeat leading with the left foot. Move through this sequence 2 – 4 times.

This isn't about quantity, more about a slow gathering and drawing inwards of the mind. The challenge is to go at a pace that facilitates this space.

Consolidate your will. **Salabhasana (Locust pose):**

Feel firm in all that supports the guide ropes of the back of the body. Stability through all our panels gives our upright self a chance to stand taller, stronger and with more grace in all of life's aliveness.

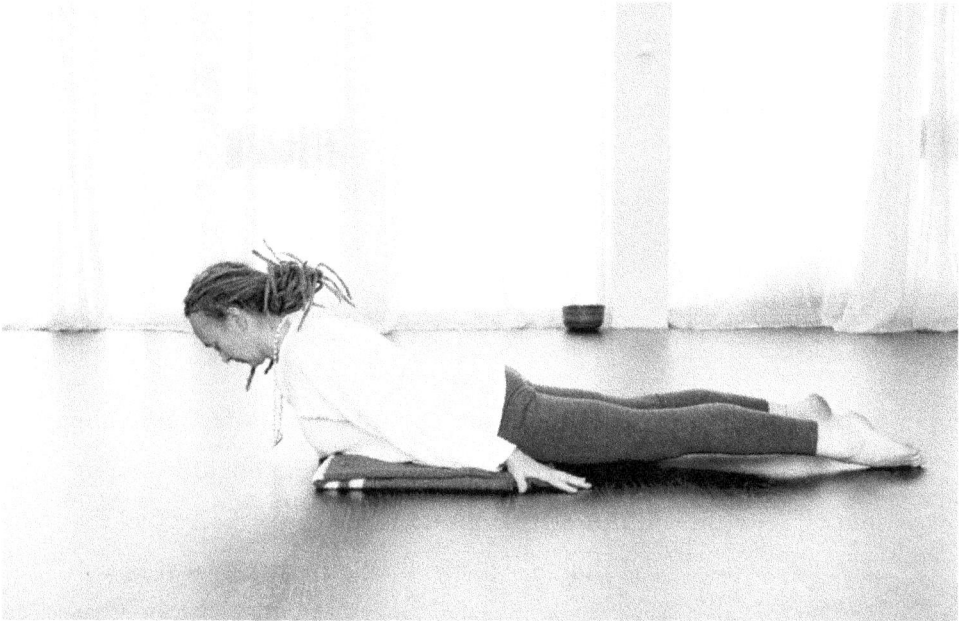

Come down to lying on your belly with your palms on the floor either side of your hips, forehead on the ground.

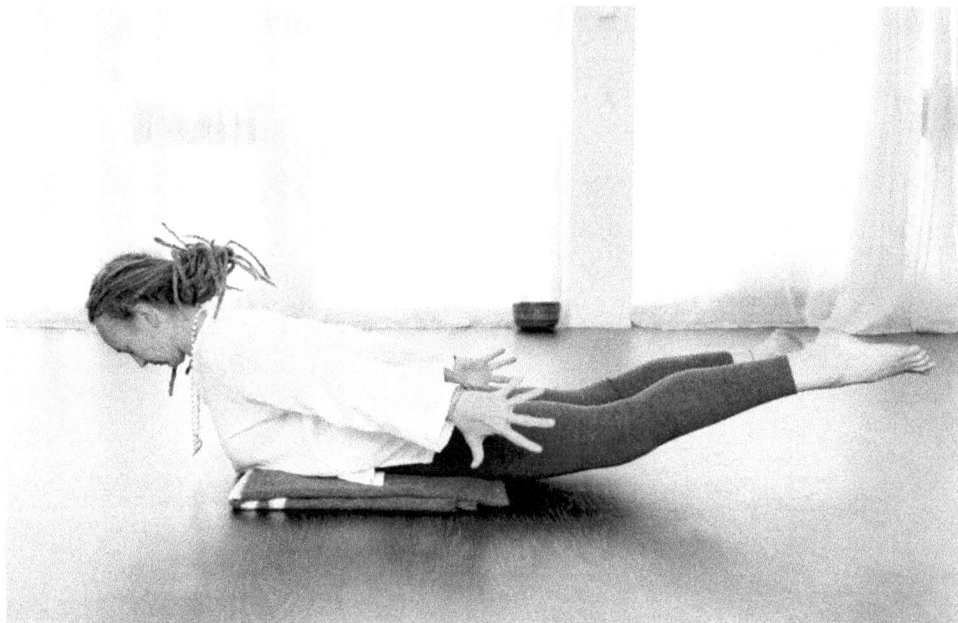

Exhale, press the palms, pubic bone and tops of feet into the ground to anchor you, raise the head, neck and shoulders, being sure to keep the chin in. Lift from the back of the body, feel the clearway between the shoulder blades as the chest comes forward.

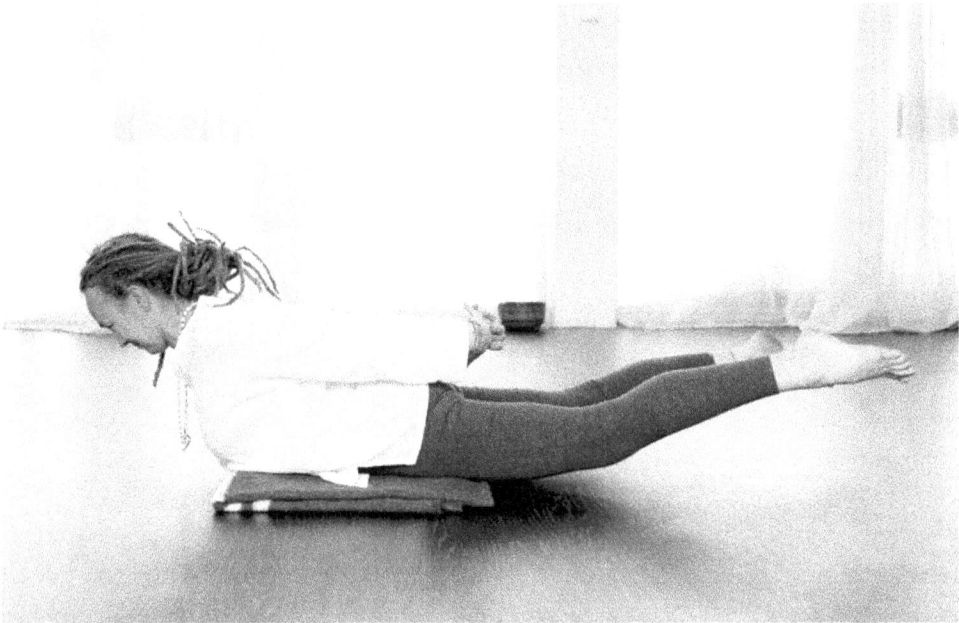

Deepen the pose by interlacing the hands behind the back if comfortable for the shoulders.

Hold for 2 – 4 breaths then lower to the mat. If you're feeling strong, raise the legs as well as the torso.

Repeat 2 – 4 times. Rest in child's pose.

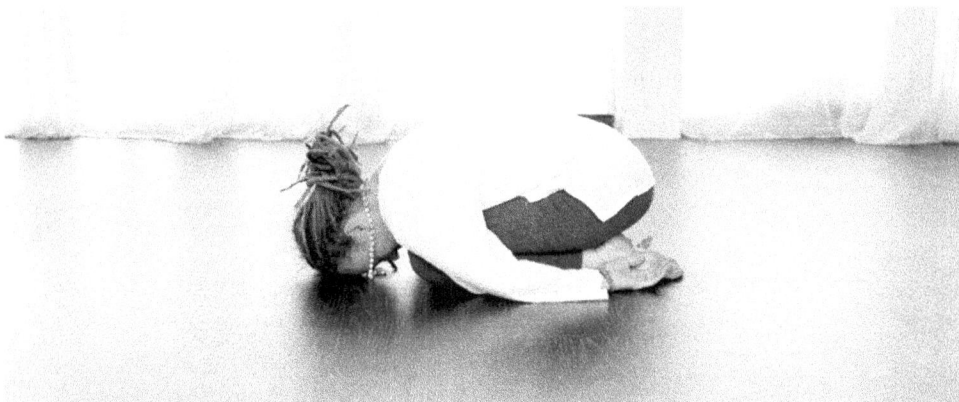

Disperse your excess.
Bharadvajasana (Seated spinal twist):

The soft twisting practices all serve to disperse accumulations. These may be physical or emotional for one will give rise to the other. We don't actively let go, it just happens as we begin to understand the lessons. The new perspective that surrender offers enables us to make the changes that we need to make in order to align with our purpose.

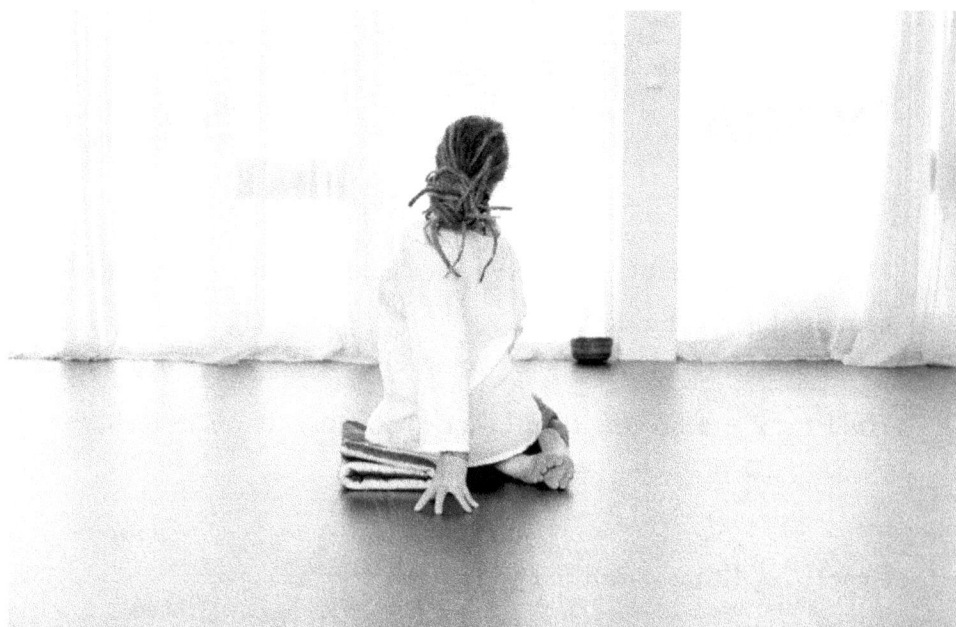

Roll up to a kneeling position. Drop your hips to the right and rest them on the floor. Bring your folded legs a little to the left of you, just outside your left hip.

Exhale and twist to the right. Use your hands as a gentle assist.

Inhale and lengthen your spine, leaning back and opening your chest a little.

Exhale to de-rotate the head and neck (look for a very sweet feeling of upper back and neck release here — divine).

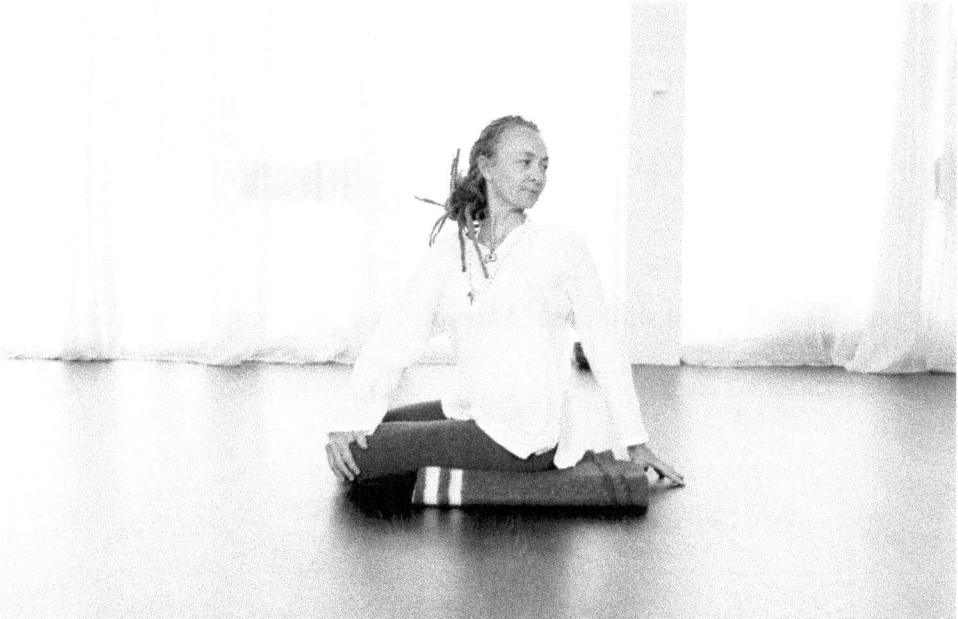

Hold here for a couple of breaths. Inhale and return to your centre. Repeat on the opposite side.

If this feels too tight for you, sit on a blanket to raise the seat.

The view from here. Setu Bandha (Supported backbend):

Towards the end of last week's sequence we spent time in a supported backbend pose over a blanket stock or bolster. Turn to page 55 and repeat for 1 – 3 minutes.

Roll out to the side and come up to an easy cross leg position and drop the torso forward to unfasten any gathering in the lower back. Repeat with the opposite crossover of the legs.

Breath yourself home.
Nadi Shodhana (Alternate Nostril Breathing):

Return to sitting in your chair or remain on the floor in an easy seated position of which there are as many variations as there are people.

Do alternate nostril breathing for 3 – 8 minutes.
As practiced in Week 1, Page 19.

Rest and integrate. Legs up the wall:

Finish the sequence with 5 – 10 minutes of resting your legs up the wall. Notice your breath and how the belly drops back towards the spine with each letting go.

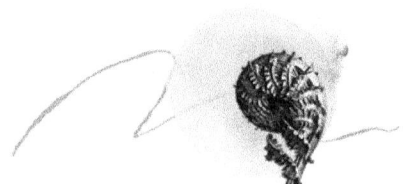

The Places In between

*"The moment a child is born, the mother is also born.
She never existed before. The woman existed, but the mother,
never. A mother is something absolutely new."*

— Osho

The shape of motherhood in its early weeks can bring us into an unfamiliar relationship with space and stillness. We can't get up when we want to because someone has fallen asleep on our chest. We can't make tea or take a phone call because someone else is demanding our attention, and both of our hands. We can't shower, brush our teeth or even go to the toilet alone anymore.

Too often we believe that the dense and dizzy blur of 'doing' is the only way for us to become, however, many of the external things that defined us have suddenly become obsolete. When we can no longer reference ourselves by the familiar landmarks we can feel lost in the unexplored hum of our inner world.

These long days in small company, the dark tired nights that follow, can make us feel like we are treading water, doing nothing, going nowhere. Not becoming.

The world around us is still filled with uprising and creativity, however our lessons right now are found in stillness, patience, allowance and compassion. We are incubating below the surface, we are resting and rounding out a shift in our lives that cannot be underestimated. In many ways we have to re-learn how to be in the quiet of ourselves so that we can better integrate and readjust after the bloom of birth.

The babymoon stretches time to give you every opportunity to come home to this place of non-doing and allowing to be. It is almost as if we are halfway over a bridge, neither here nor there, not quite who we were, not quite who we will become. This place of duality is where you gather who you are now, in light of all that has shifted in your world, doing so to discover what the world is asking of you now.

Just as the moon grows full then dissolves into darkness, its radiance dependant on the culmination of all its stages, we must learn to honour the call to rest that this time brings so our radiance can return when the spirit is ready.

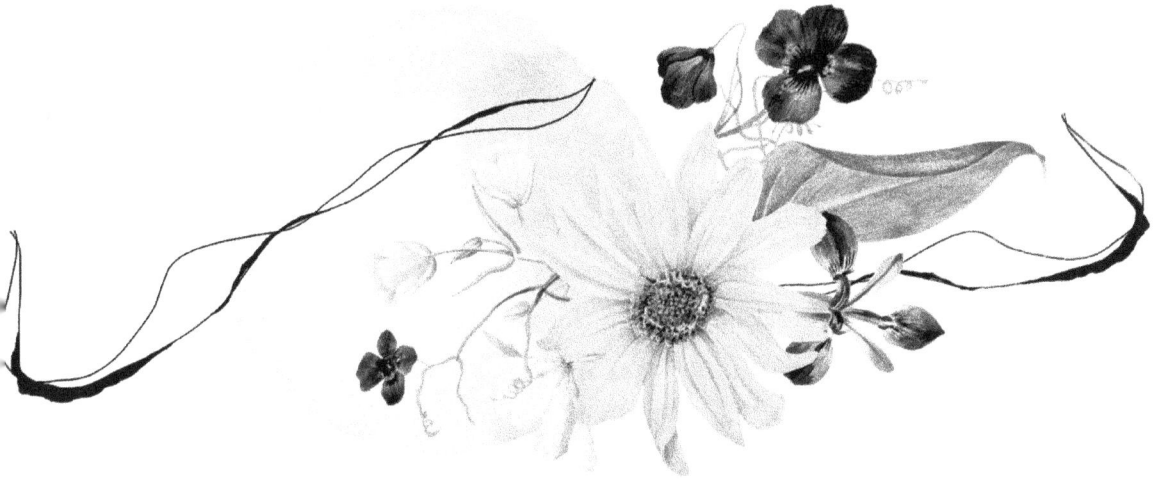

Start where you are. **Supported Setu Bandha (backbend):**

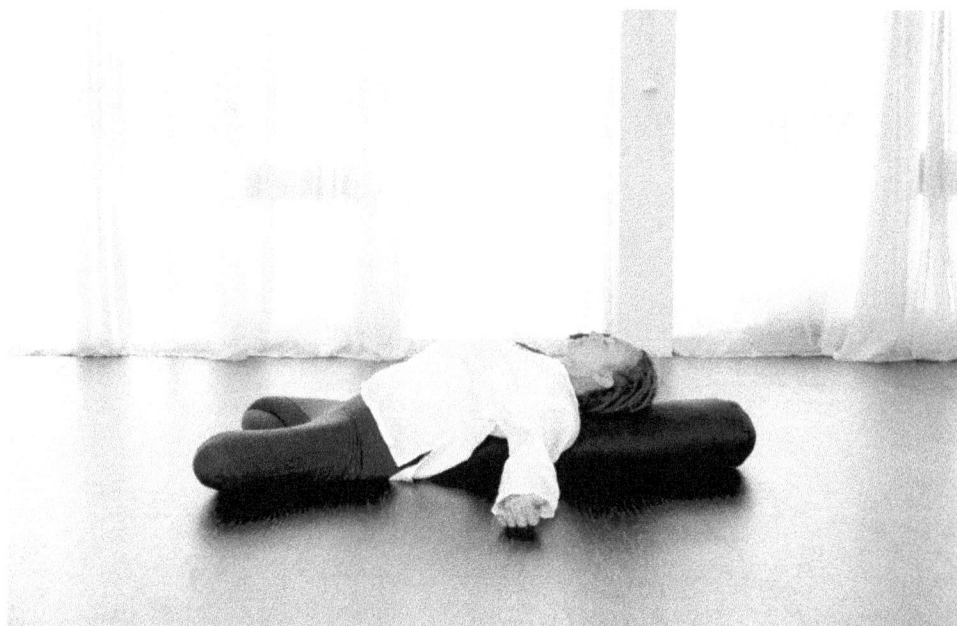

Use folded blankets or a bolster if you are lucky enough to have one, to build a support under your spine and the back of the head. With your buttocks resting on the ground, lay yourself back over your supports, extending your arms out to the sides of the body.

This pose must feel comfortable and supported.

Begin to take control of your breath, to attend to that which arises in one breath cycle and no more. Lean your attention towards the exhalation, practicing emptying the breath all the way into the still point at its end. Pause here. Let the inhalation come naturally, filling the body from the belly to the diaphragm to the collarbones.

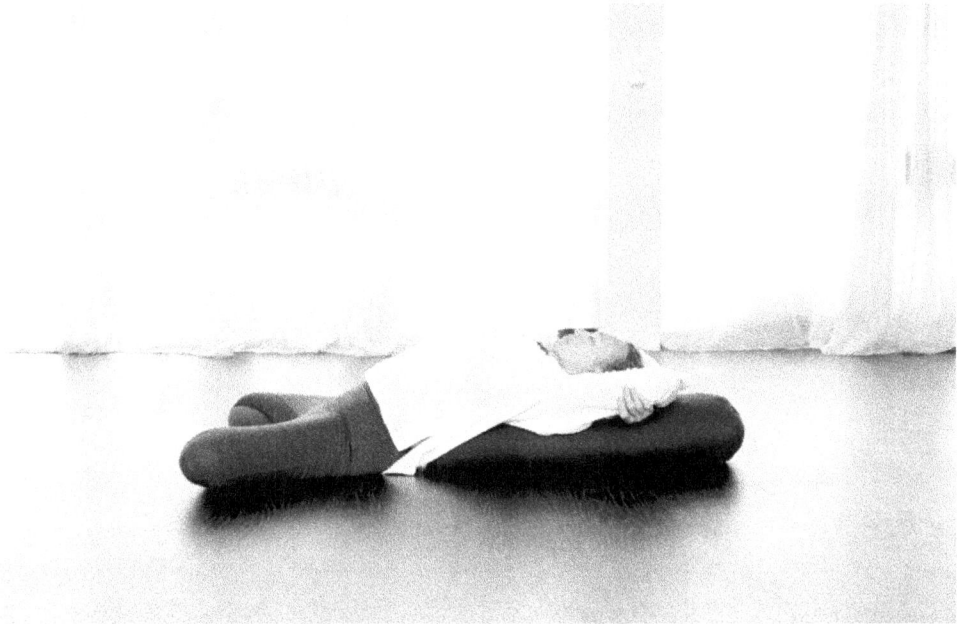

Allow the exhalation to slowly grow in length. Raise the arms overhead to rest the forearms on your blanket stack or bolster if there is space in the shoulders.

Stay with this practice for 3 – 5 minutes.

To release, roll out to the side and come into child's pose.

Fortify what you can't see. **Bhujangasana (Cobra pose):**

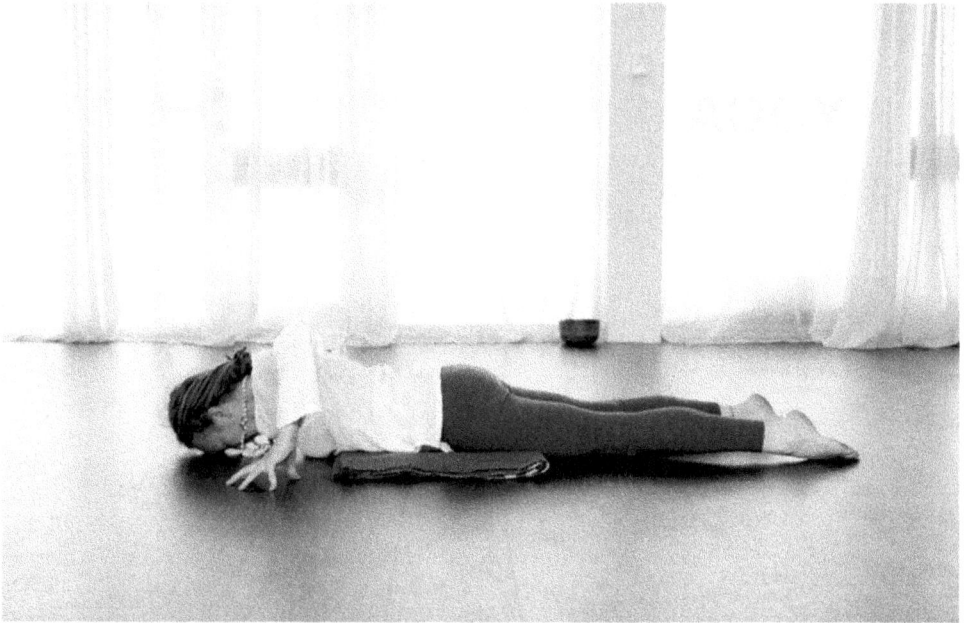

Lie on the floor on your belly with your feet in line with your hips, the front of the feet spreading on the mat. Lift your pubic bone a little towards your navel so it feels like you are trying to lift the lower belly away from the floor. To create the foundation for the chest work, place your fingertips on the floor outside your mat and level with your shoulders. Your bent elbows are reaching towards the ceiling, your forehead is on the floor.

* If you find lying on the belly uncomfortable for your full breasts use the spinal toning all-fours asana from week 3.

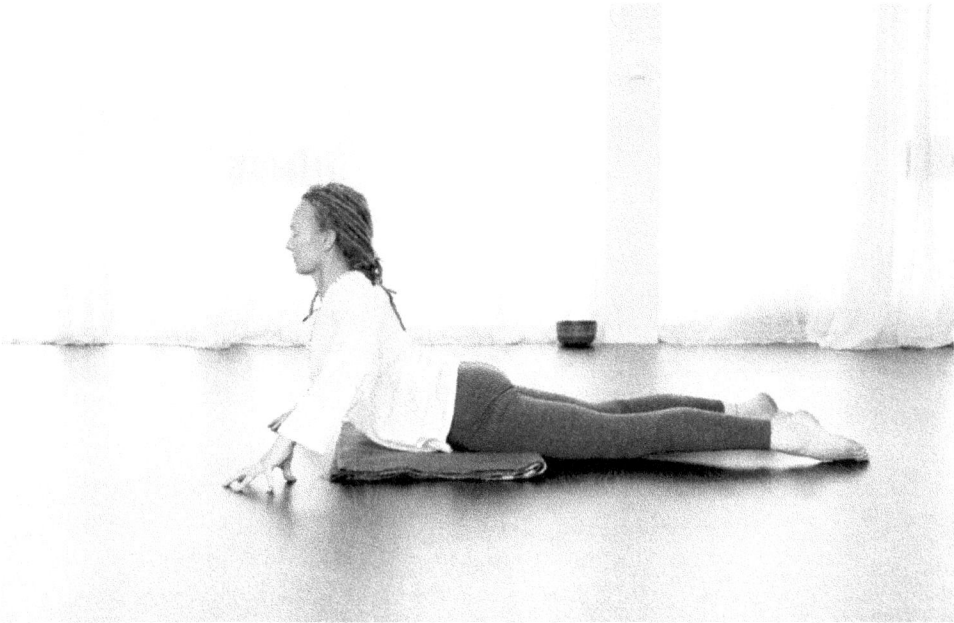

Inhale, press the fingers down and raise the torso feeling the spinal muscles spreading.

Exhale and lower back to your starting position.

Repeat this rolling for 4 – 8 times, holding for a few breaths on the last one.

This pose can be repeated for another round or two if it feels beneficial. It is strengthening by nature and releasing by stealth. Your shoulder blades are the measure of the chest softening here so look for a feeling of descent in them, like they hug the back rather than ride up to the ears.

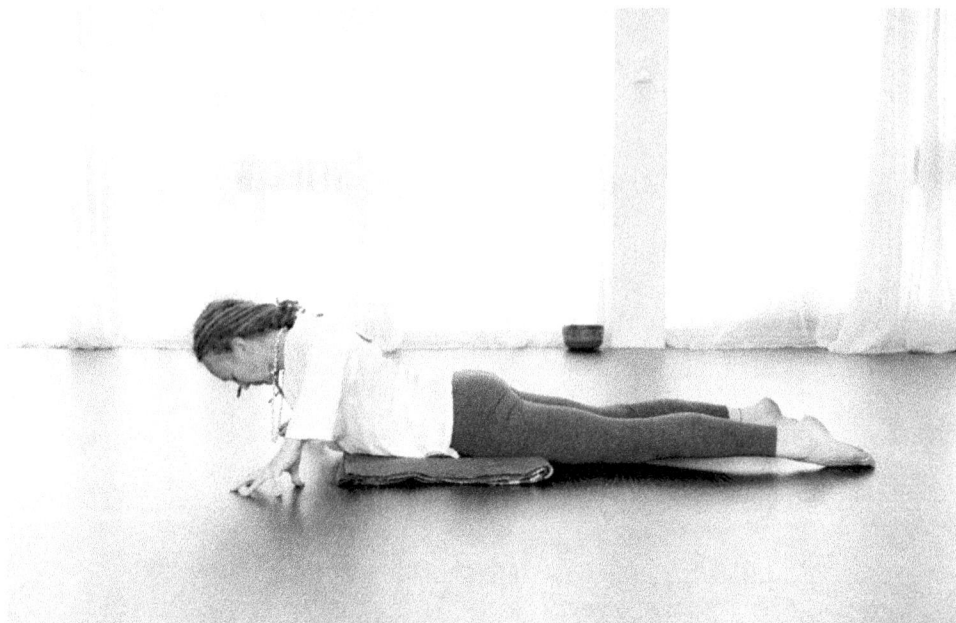

Only go as high as the spine allows for an even curve in its length.

Press yourself back to child's pose for a few breaths before lifting to downward facing dog pose.

Wrap yourself around your possibilities. **Parivrtta Parsvakonasana variation (High lunge with a twist):**

Inquire into the framework of the pillar of the spine as you navigate your way around its bones. Twist from your inside out. Honour first what's below and beneath.

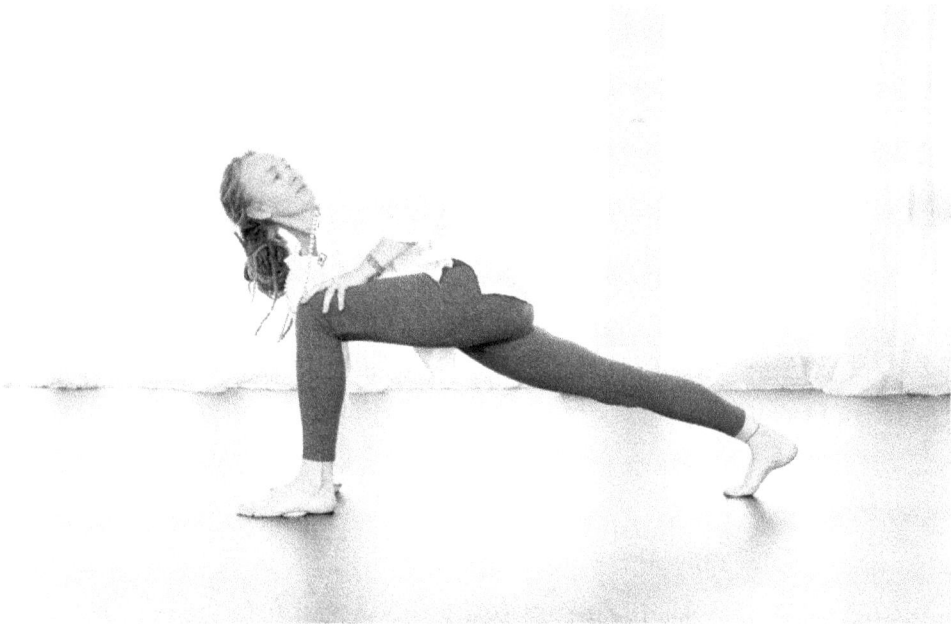

From your downward-facing dog pose, step your right foot forward to a high-lunge base. Looking down at your hands, keep the left hand where it is and bring the right hand to the right knee.

Exhale and twist your torso to the right.

Inhale and raise the right arm to the vertical if there's space in the shoulder.

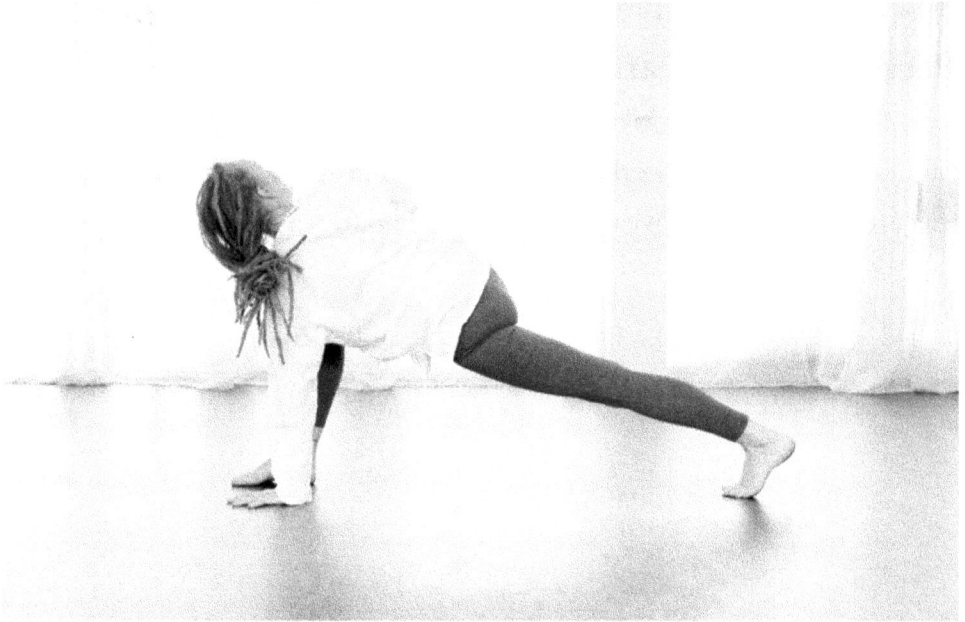

As you hold here for a few breaths feel the turn of the pose rising from the navel as it spins itself to the right. Lean back a little, let it take you.

Exhale and release the pose and step back to downward-facing dog for the opposite side.

* Simplify the shape by placing your back knee on the ground.

Spiral in. **Prasarita Padottanasana (Wide leg forward fold):**

This sweet, supported forward fold gives a chance for the uterus, bowel and bladder to reverse their downdraft and fall towards the base of the diaphragm instead. This gives them renewed circulation and much needed decompression. The lower the head the slower the breath and the more soft the mind becomes.

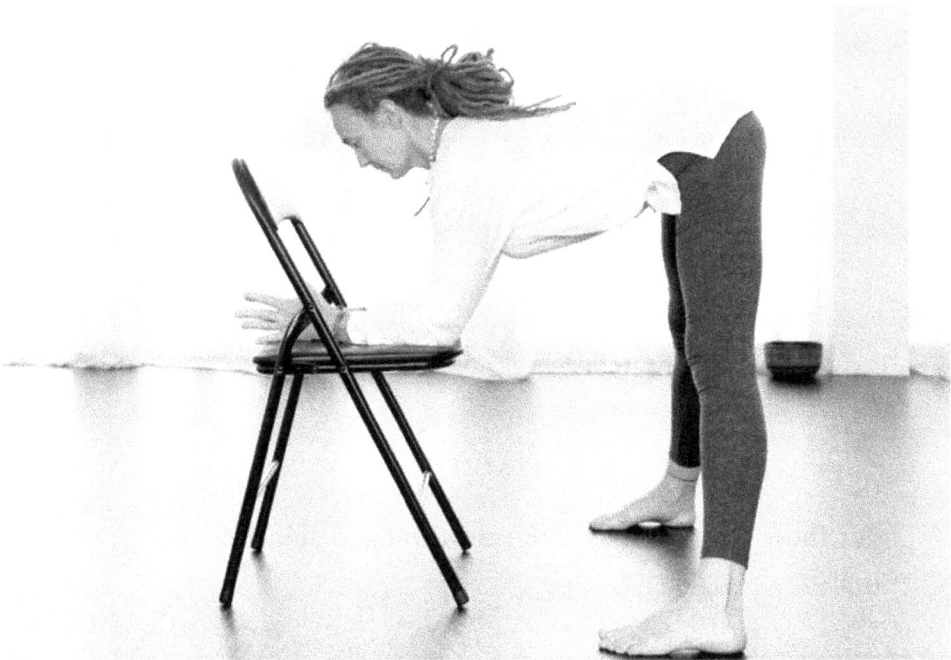

Come to standing, widening the feet to double shoulder width or a little wider and have a chair in front of you with the seat facing towards you. Place your hands on your hips and look upwards, creating a sweet standing backbend shape.

Exhale and fold forward bringing your palms, forearms or forehead to the chair seat.

With deep breaths hold here for 1 – 3 minutes working on lengthening your spine — even if that means the knees have to soften a little.

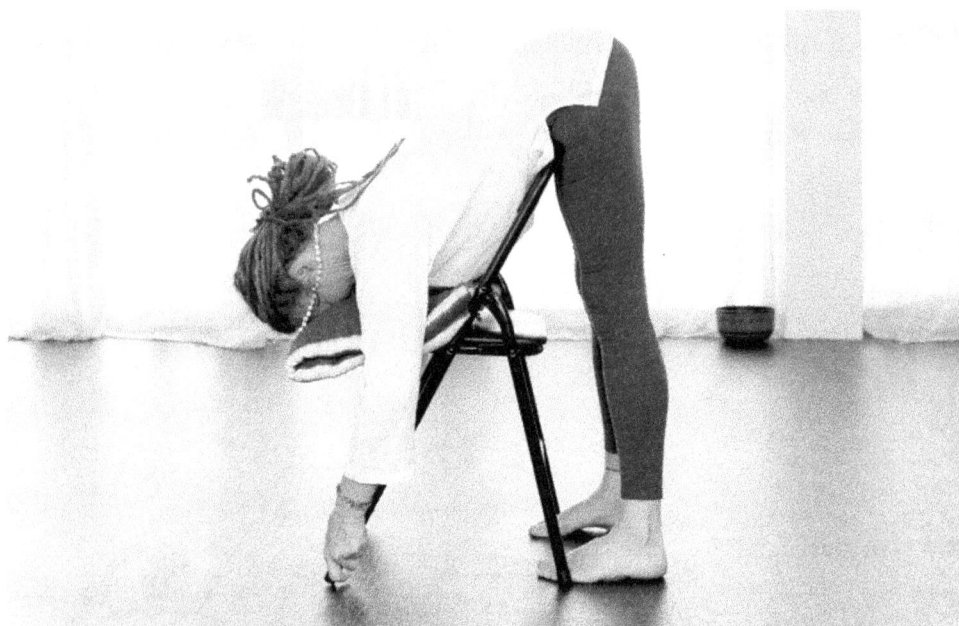

For those with a little more hamstring and spinal flexibility, try this deeper version.

Turn the chair around so the back rest faces towards you and place a blanket or towel on the seat to support your head. It can be beneficial to place a towel or such over the back rest so it's soft on your belly.

Fold forward with the backrest of the chair at the crease of the legs.

Blow on the coals of the heart.
Supported Setu Bandha (Bridge Pose):

This is a slightly different version of the supported backbend we have been working on and offers a deeper aspect to be discovered. If you aren't sure, return to the supported backbend we did at the beginning of this practice, otherwise...

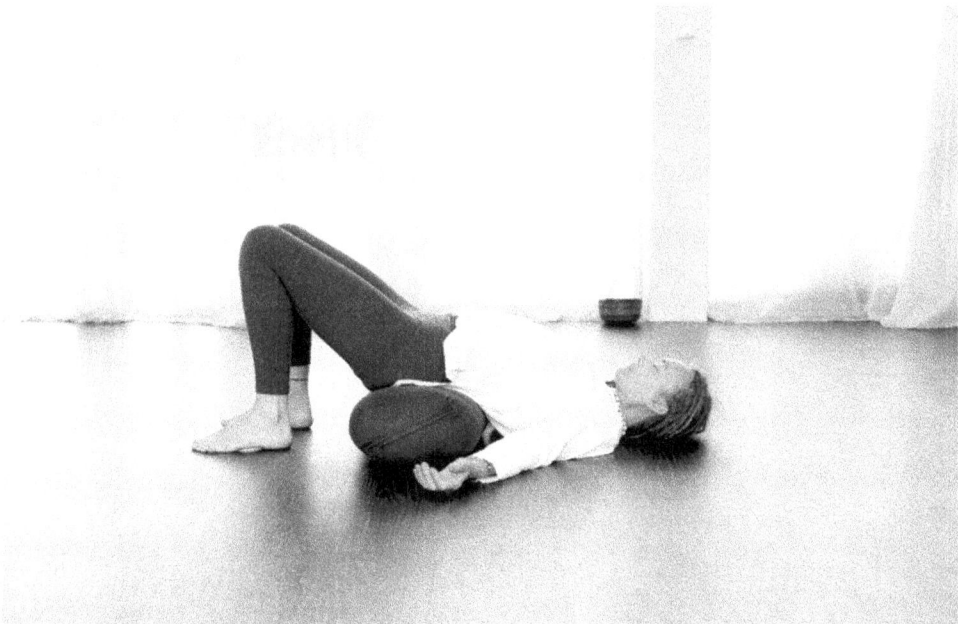

Take the bolster or blanket stack parallel to your sacrum (rather than perpendicular to it). Roll yourself backwards over the support, finding it nestling into your mid/lower back. Your head shoulders and buttocks are all on the floor. Extend your arms out to the sides on the upper side of the support.

Stay here for 1 – 3 minutes.

* *If it feels too strong, lower the support height to a single folded towel or blanket. If that's not possible, put a cushion or other rise under the back of the head to reduce the thoracic curve.*

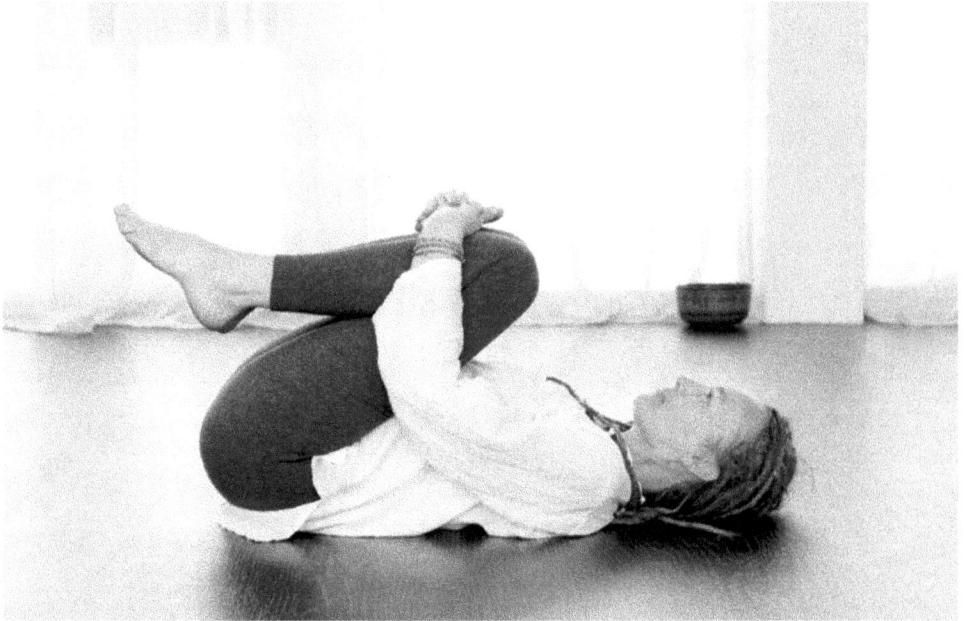

Lift your hips and remove the support. Hug your knees into your chest to release the back. Rock a little side to side. Stay while it feels good.

Going deeper. **Reclined Rajakapotasana (Pigeon Pose):**

You may know this as a back-release pose or 'thread the needle'. This pose actions the channels in the body most closely related to the large intestine meridian having the wonderful effect of a downward, outward, letting go sigh. Use this pose to ground the stillness you have been cultivating.

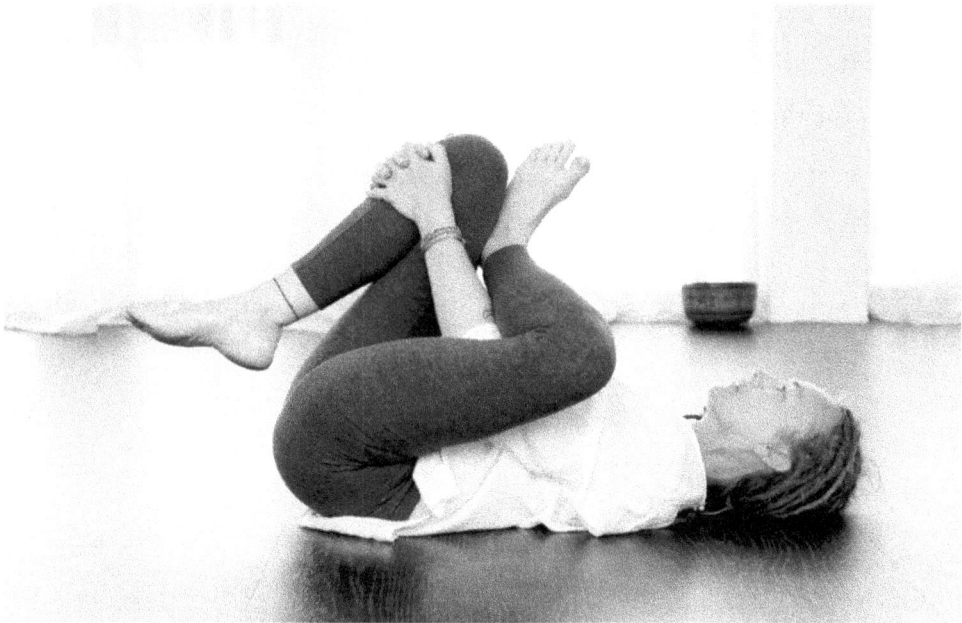

From lying on your back, bend both your knees bringing the soles of the feet to the floor and knees to the ceiling. Cross your right ankle over your left knee and draw the left knee towards the chest until you feel a warming in the right hip.

You can hold the left shinbone through the window of the right leg, hold the back of the left knee, or use a strap to fill the space between the hands and the knee. It's about your hip not the interlace of your hands or how close the non working leg is to the body.

Hold here with deep slow breaths, balancing the weight on the centre of the sacrum for 1 – 3 minutes before releasing and setting up for the opposite side.

Taking it all in.
Supta Paschimottanasana (Forward Fold):

Fold unfold, squeeze release, it's the rhythmic law under which we are all students. Just like in childbirth, learning to accept that for every expansion there is an equal and opposite contraction helps us build trust in all the rhythms of our aliveness.

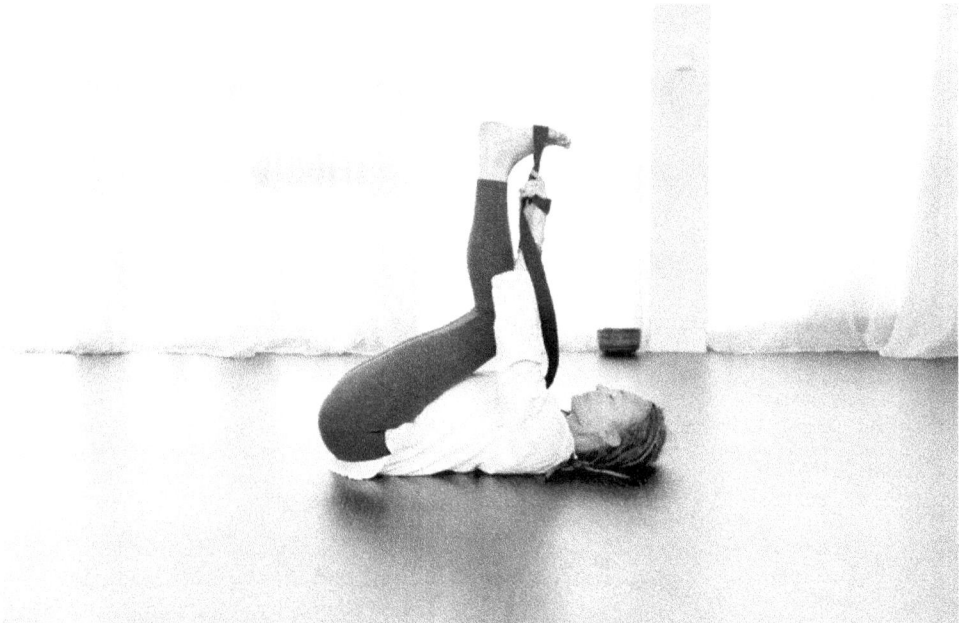

From lying on your back bring both knees to the chest and hug them in. This is Upanasana, the Great Neutralizer. Just stay here if its honesty is calling you.

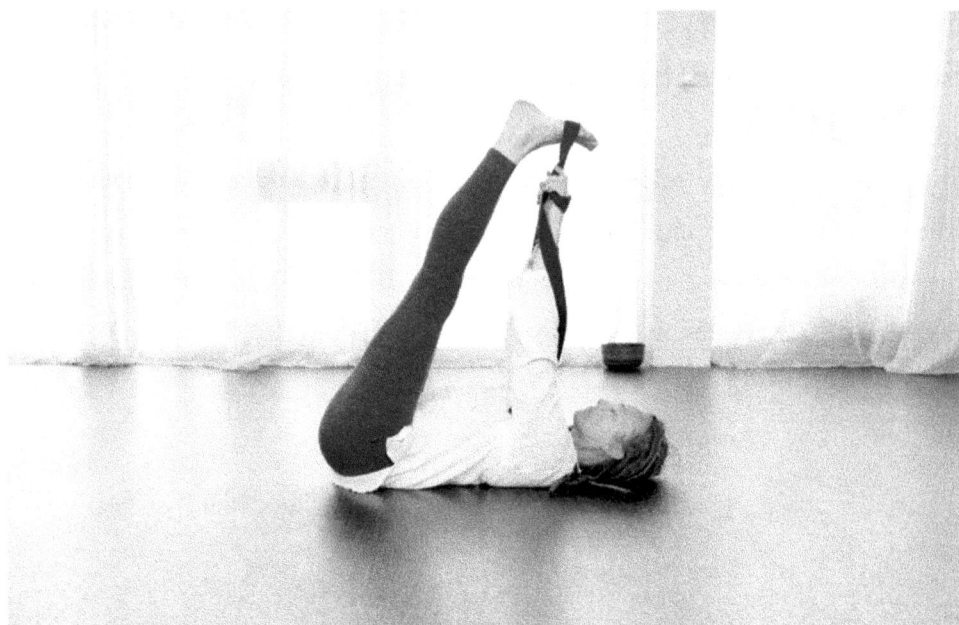

To extend the pose take both legs into the vertical placing a strap around the balls of the feet such that the weight of the strap catches the weight of the legs and all falls into grace and effortless balance at the sacrum and lower back. You've got this.

If the legs do not straighten it's still the pose. Feet over the hips is the only navigation required.

Rest. **Its dividends are greater than you think. Sivasana:**

3 – 5 minutes minimum.

When the internal light is low and the times feel challenging without end, the answer to all you seek is behind your eyes and in the spaces between your breaths.

In this pose you are lying flat on your back on the floor. Bring a soft support under the head if needed. Here we take deep rest. Never, ever skip this part of your practice — particularly if it's new to you or it feels foreign. Set a timer somewhere nearby and hand over to that time with all that you have. Everything, and I mean everything — except a waking baby — will wait. I promise.

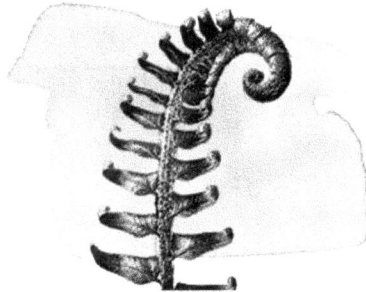

The Emerging

*"You are a spring breeze just beginning to take flight.
You are the breath of God (Self, Guru), the cradle of light.
You are formless, boundless potential as great as the sky all
packed in a body that itself creates life."*

— Cristen Rogers

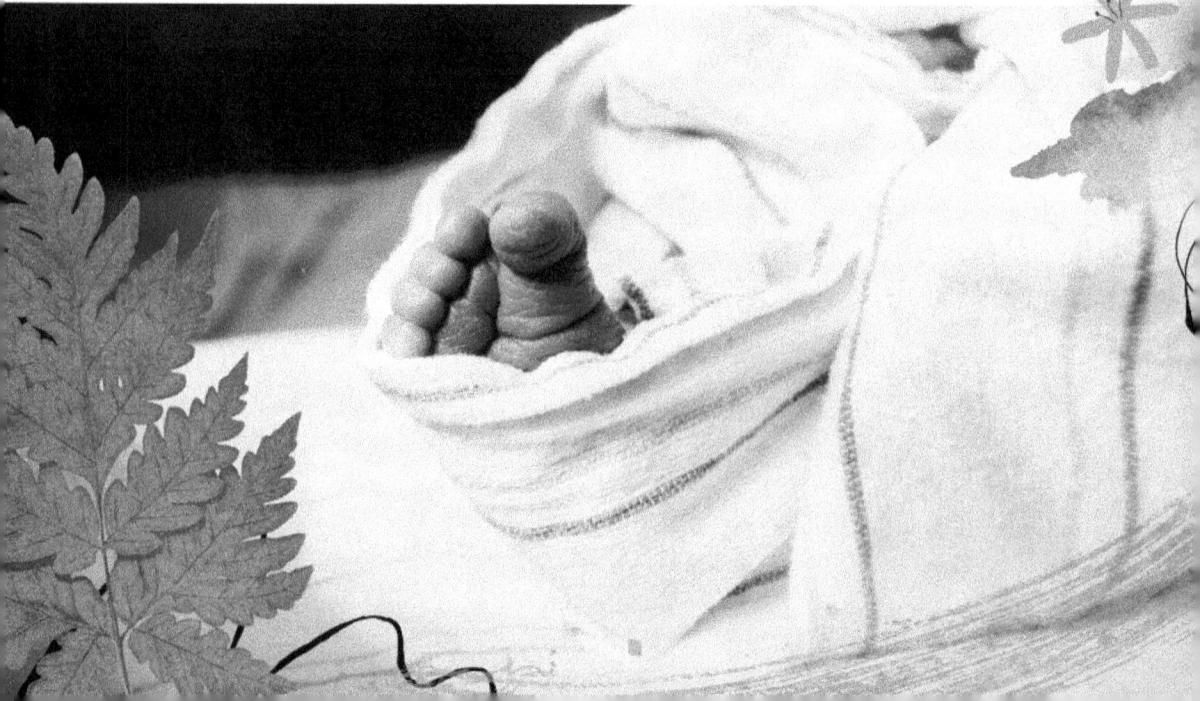

Our transition to Motherhood represents one of the greatest leaps we take as women. At around 6 weeks post birth you are, for the most part, healed from the physical journey of birthing. You have had time, space and opportunity to be present in your new role and its various presentations. You have talked and cried and laughed and loved, and a sense of who you are becoming is beginning to emerge with more clarity. Motherhood is a watershed, a resonant song from a strata of your being that you are only beginning to touch. Motherhood is standing tall in the call of your Soul.

The soft, gentle work of your yoga practice continues tirelessly, even when you are not on the mat, helping you find the way to the insights, dreams and visions that are trying to come to the surface right now. You are living among a short and profoundly magical time and everything calls you to breathe yourself into the fullness of this new version of life. While it may be easy to pretend that we are fine, unaffected even by the life changing events of the last few weeks, it is far richer to lean into what you came to know of yourself in the process. This is heart felt navigation and it's the most honest way forward from here.

Are you honouring what is trying to grow?

When you breathe life into your whispers, all of your being rejoices, you become full and luminous, living in union with what you are being gently nudged towards.

Seek the woman that is trying to live through you now, she is your new life's work and she will continue to grow to a round and full octave.

Tell your deepest Self you are here to listen.
Bow down to the one within.
Give yourself the gift of your Soul.

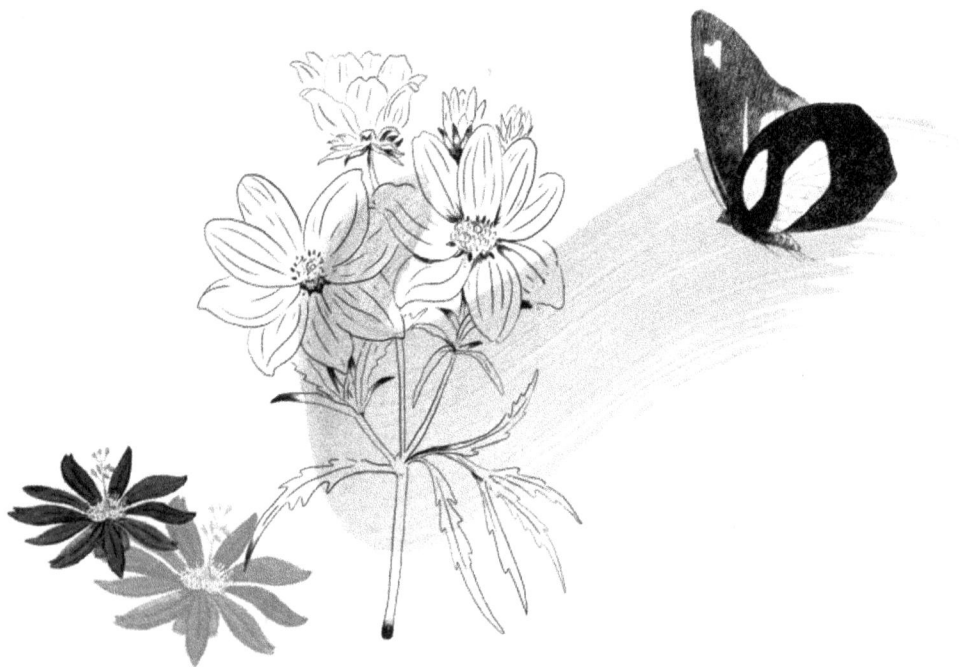

Take stock. **Supta Hasta Padangusthasana (Reclining hand to big toe pose):**

This sequence is old, unchanged and so very sweet. You have nothing to accomplish here other than to take the shape and turn the Being of your action inward.

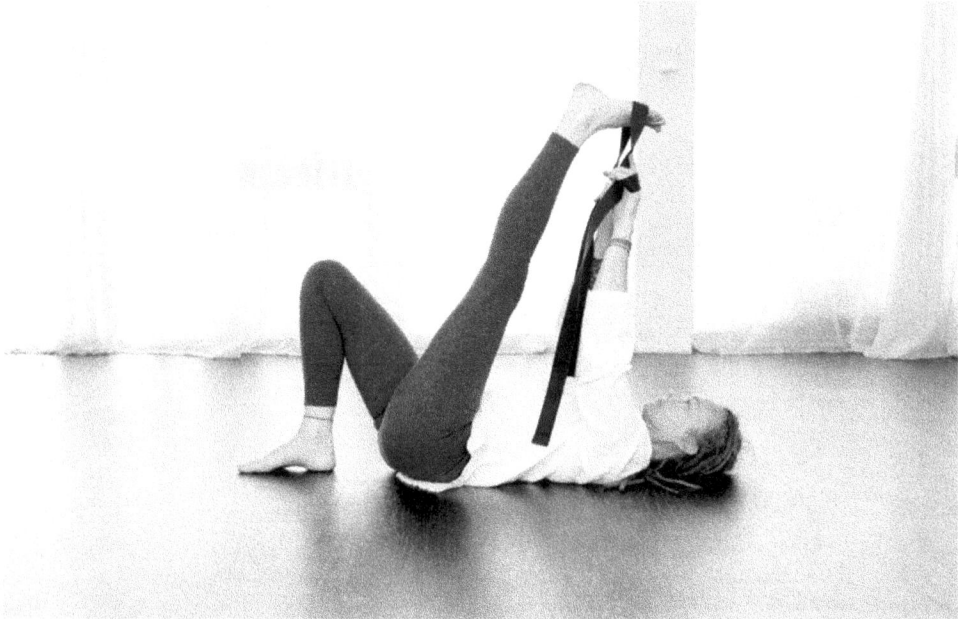

Start lying on your back. Soles of the feet on the floor, both knees bent. Bring the right knee towards the chest and loop a strap over the ball of the foot.

Exhale and straighten or half straighten the leg towards the ceiling flexing the foot strongly. Keep your chin moving towards your chest. Soften your shoulders.

Feel your centre as you draw the pubis a little towards the navel.
Reach out from here along the line of the raised leg towards the
heel.

Hold here for 5 – 10 breaths.

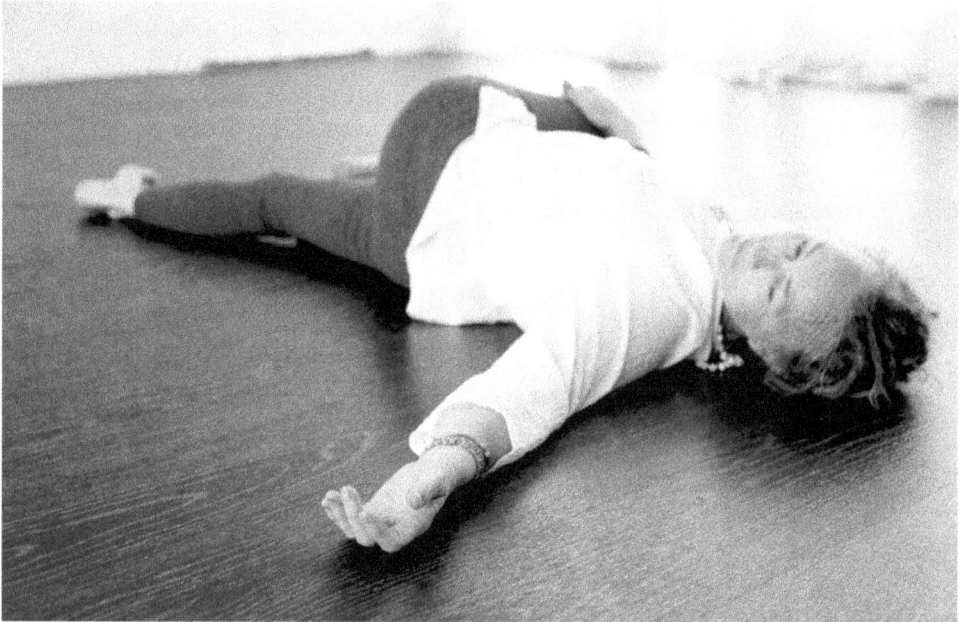

To release the pose, straighten the left bent leg along the floor,
bend the right knee and cross it over the left. Use the left hand to
take the knees across the body into a floor twist.

Hold here for 3 – 5 breaths.

Repeat the sequence on the opposite side.

Tuning spinal resonance.
Supported Setu Bandha (Bridge pose):

See Week 3, page 55 and Week 5, page 93.

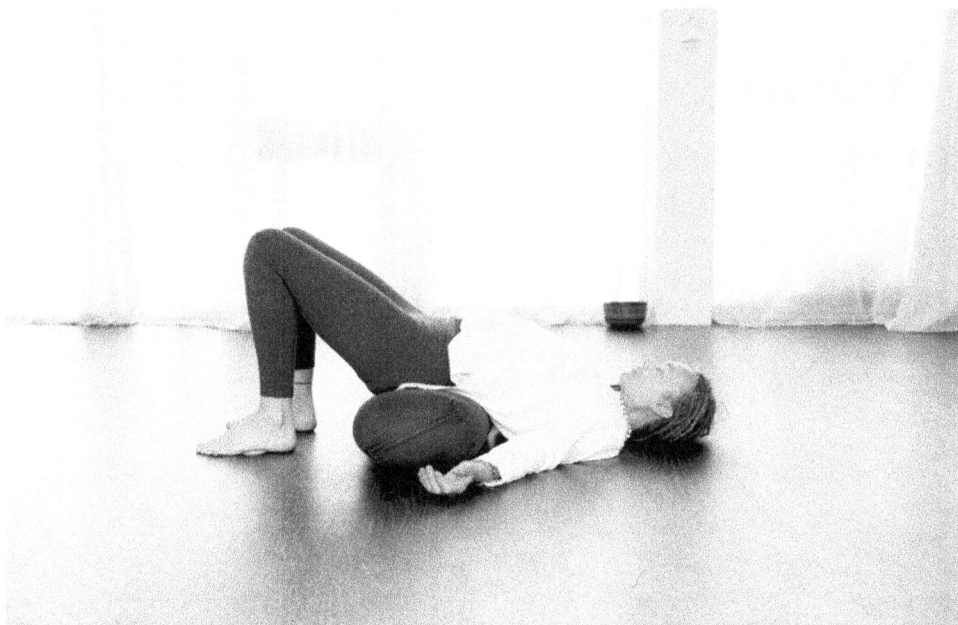

Ananda Balasana (Happy Baby Pose):

This posture gives you unbridled access to the panels of deep holding that reside in the lower back and sacrum. Like a storage silo of your secrets, your desires, your hopes — enter slowly. Breathe deeply. Be delighted.

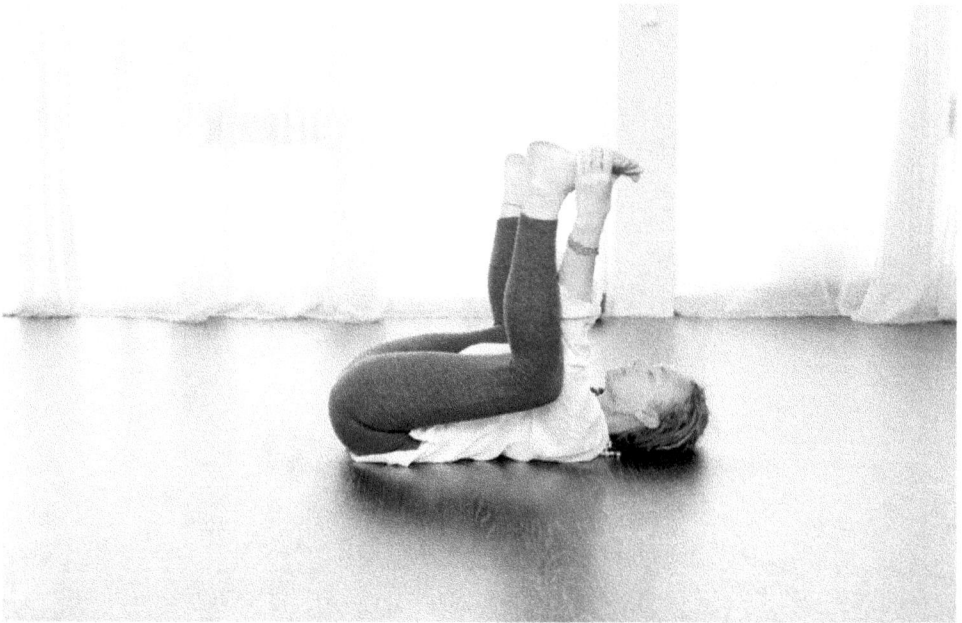

From lying on your back hug your knees towards your chest. Hold the little toe side of each foot and slowly swing the shins towards perpendicular. If the lower back or groin feels resistant, hold the tops of the shins, keep the heels low and widen the knees to the sides.

Place a cushion or folded blanket under the back of the head if the throat is over-opening.

Press the lower back and sacrum to the floor and allow the lower spine to bathe in the healing waters of the dural fluids.

This can be a big release of pelvic tension and is best not rushed.

Hold for 5 – 10 breaths.

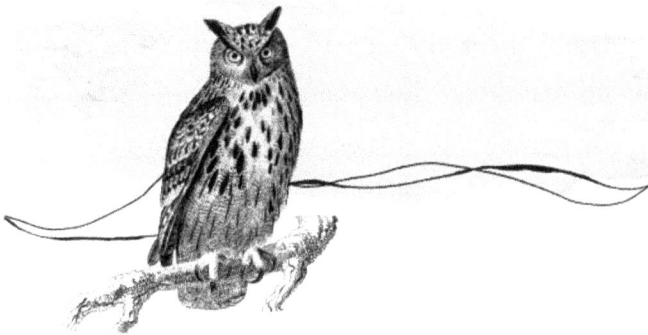

Centring thoughts and action. **Navasana (Boat pose):**

Using a rolling action we reconnect with the intelligence required to move around a soft central axis. This is something that can be lost during pregnancy and needs to be regained once we feel ready to return.

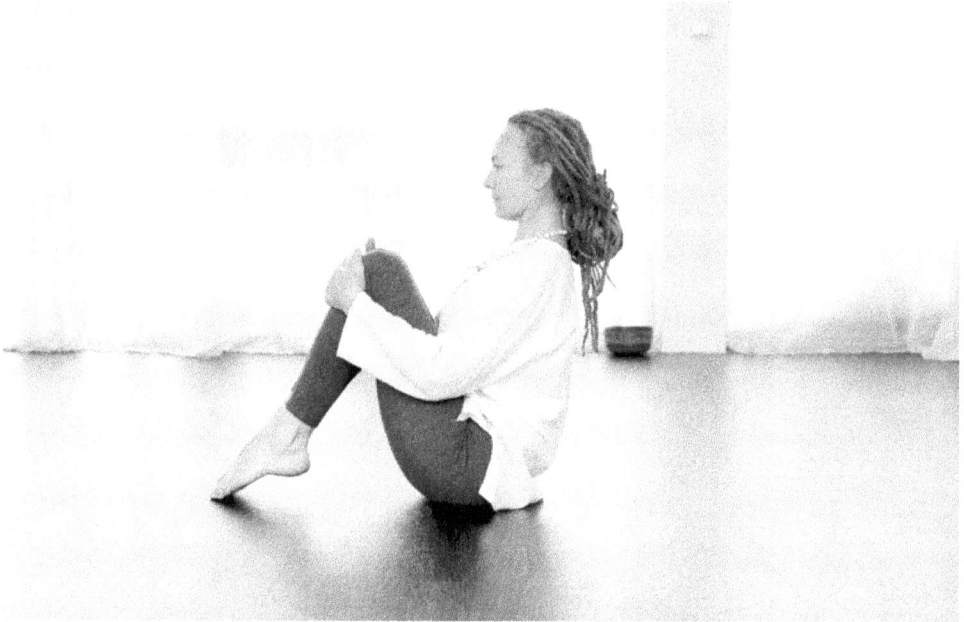

Roll yourself up to sitting with legs out long in front of you. Bend your knees and hug them in towards your chest tightly, point your toes and keep them on the floor or deepen by flexing your feet and keeping them low towards your buttocks. Try to lengthen your spine by pressing the knees away from you against the resistance of the hands around the shins — avoid rounding in the back.

Slowly release the grip of the legs and let the lower belly muscles start firing up, begin extending the hands forward of you, either side of the thighs.

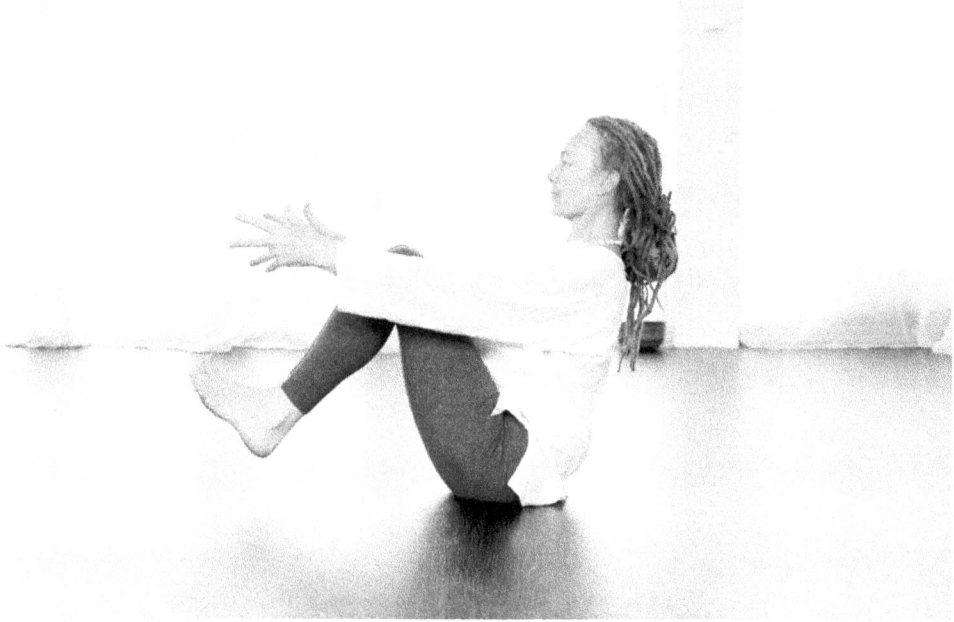

Take 3 breaths here.

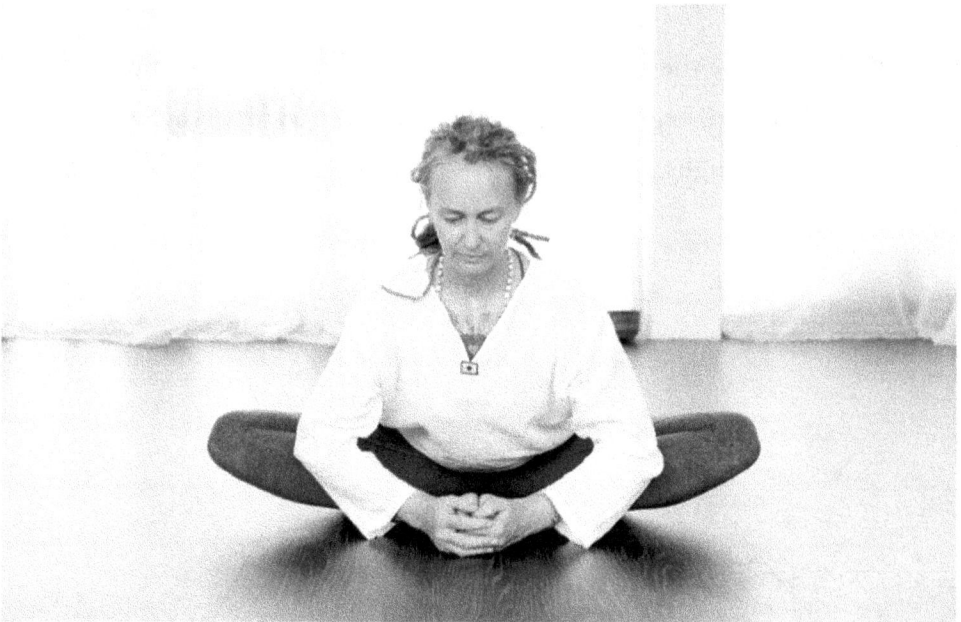

Exhale, and release the pose by returning to upright sitting and bringing the soles of the feet together, knees wide. You may like to fold forward a few degrees keeping the chest open.

Take 3 breaths here.

Exhale and return to the boat pose.

Repeat the sequence 8 – 10 times, feeling the centre develop strength and presence.

Grounding the centre down. **Malasana (Squat pose):**

This pose is the queen of the grounding currents. She places us firmly in the belly of ourselves, the deepest tones and the wildest most forbidden places — all coming to ground in the Mother energies themselves. It can be a hard place to return to after birth, sometimes an aching can rise as we begin to reconnect with the story within us. Go easy and use the props suggested until you find YOU returning to YOU.

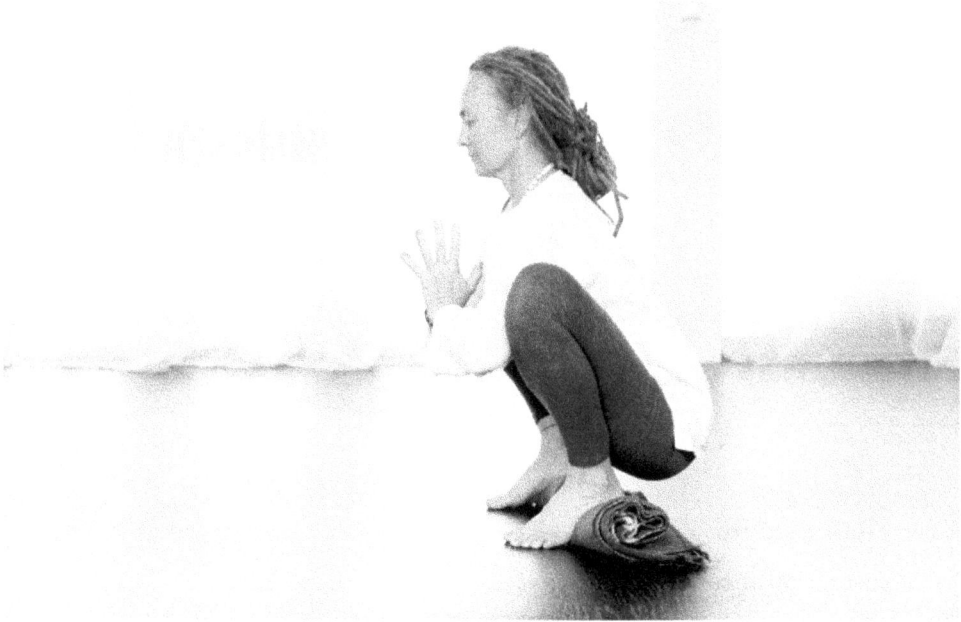

Place your feet on the floor at outer hip width and roll yourself to a squat position. If the heels don't reach the floor, roll a blanket under them to give them a little lift. If the knees are strained or there is a heaviness in the base of the body, sit on a low stool, yoga block or firm cushion to support your weight.

The palms of the hands are together in prayer at the chest, knees are wide. Elongate your spine by dropping your tailbone under and reaching upwards through the crown of the head.

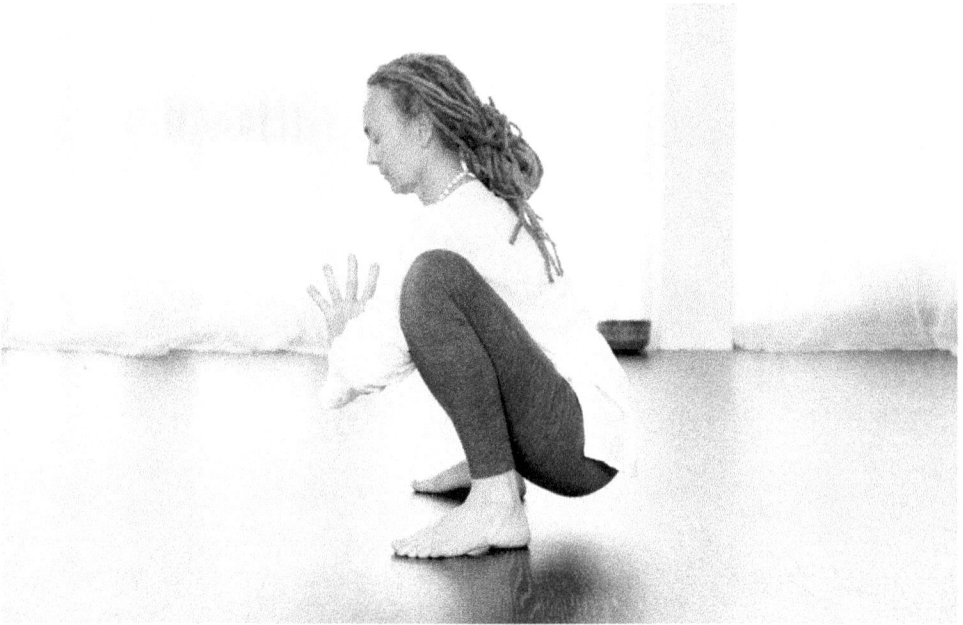

Hold here for as long as you are comfortable. A few breaths — several minutes.

To release from the pose, place your hands on the ground and slowly straighten your legs to unfold into a standing forward fold. Turn your feet parallel to one another.

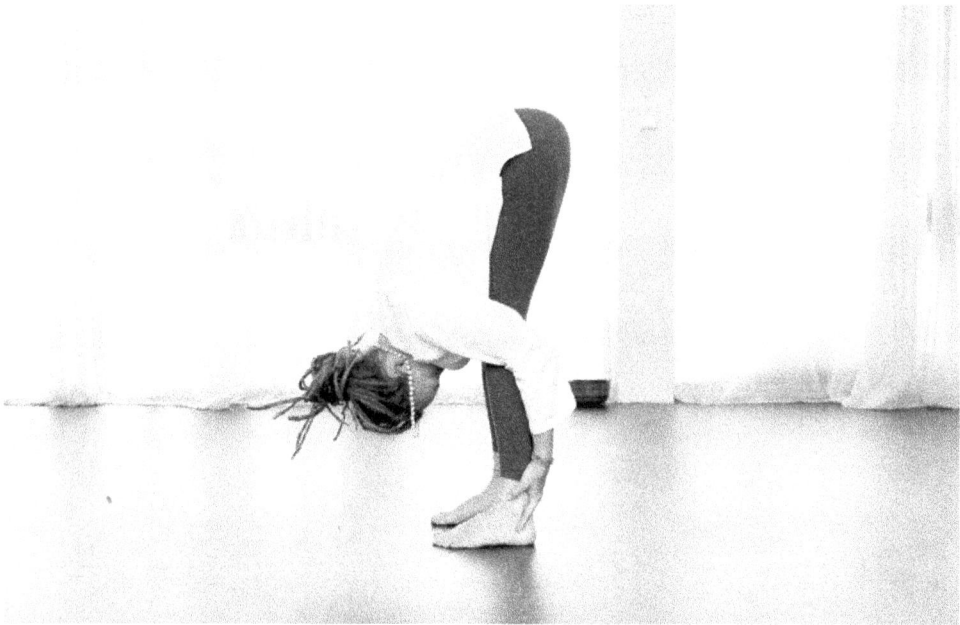

Exhale and roll up to standing.

* This pose has a caution for knee injuries. If that's you, make sure you sit on a support and go into and out of the pose slowly so you can measure its effectiveness and decide if it's best to skip it.

Stoking the fire. **Step back salutations**

See Week 4, pages 68-74.

Finish the sequence in downward-facing dog pose.

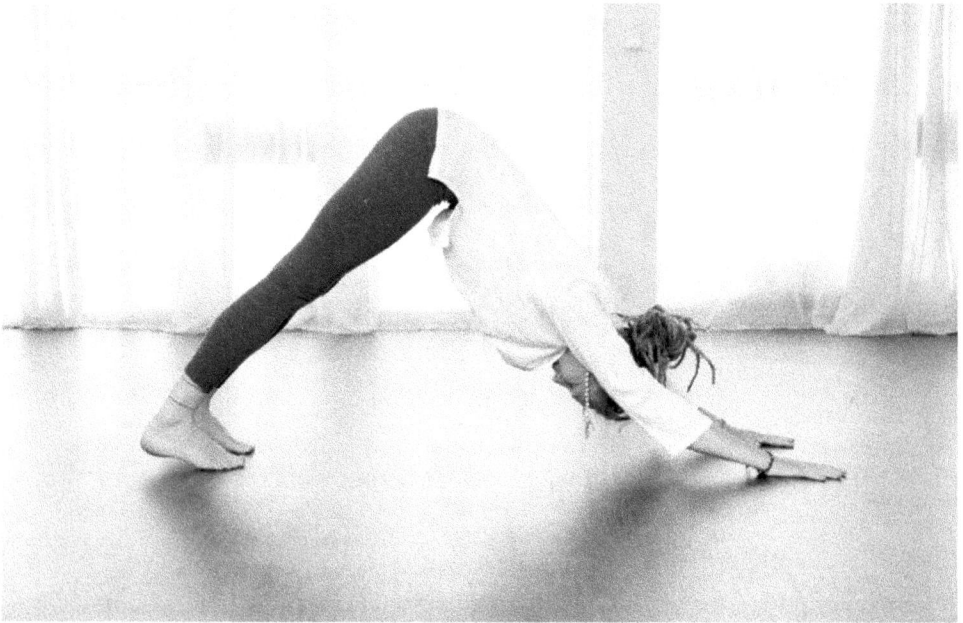

Redefining your shape. **Parsvakonasana (Side angle pose):**

So called because it lengthens and disperses the sides of the body, this master stretch really gives when it comes to the seams and everything we may be trying to hold together. Breath into its shape and let it soften any peripheral holding; open your perspective.

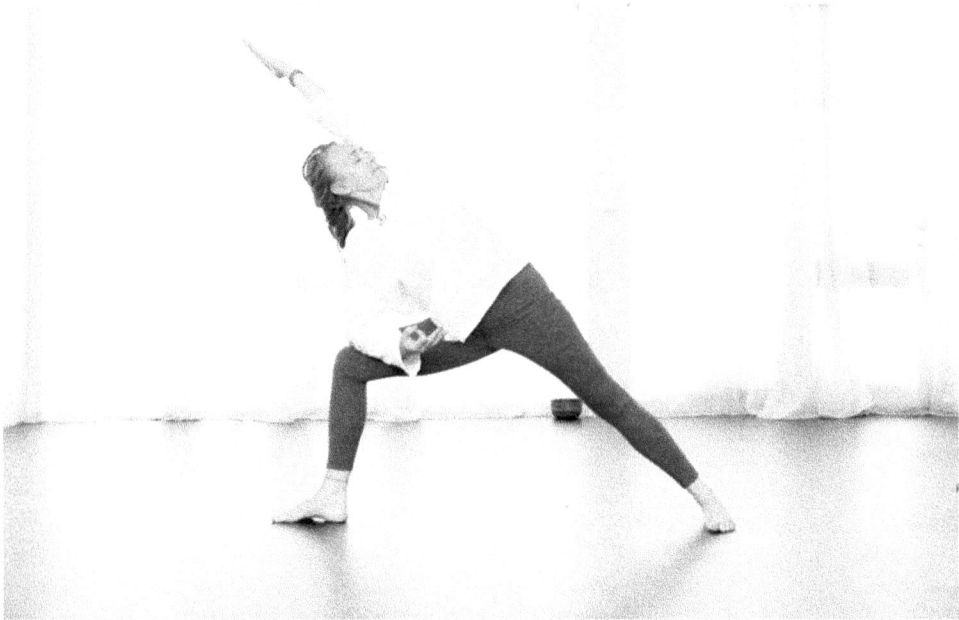

Stepping the right foot forward between the hands. Turn the back foot at 45 degrees. Bend the front right knee and place the right forearm on the thigh, left hand to the left hip.

Inhale. Lengthen the spine by pressing into the back foot and reaching towards the crown of the head.

Exhale and rotate the torso to the left, leaning back just a little.

Inhale. Raise the top arm, if comfortable, towards the ceiling and over into a lateral position.

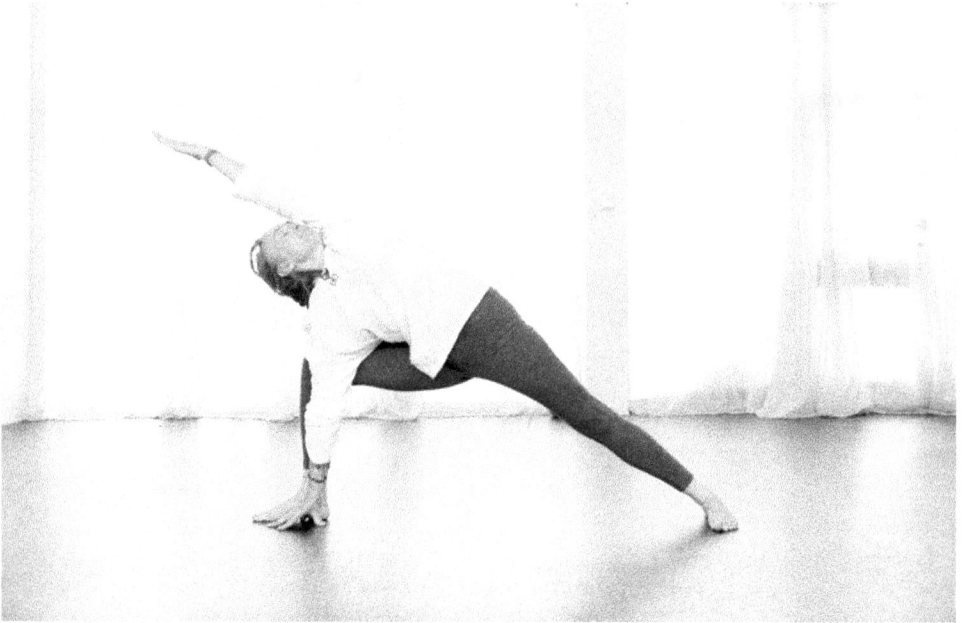

Take 3 – 5 breaths here.

Step back to downward dog and repeat on the opposite side.

Returning to silence. **Prasarita Padottanasana (Wide leg forward fold):**

See Week 5, page 91.

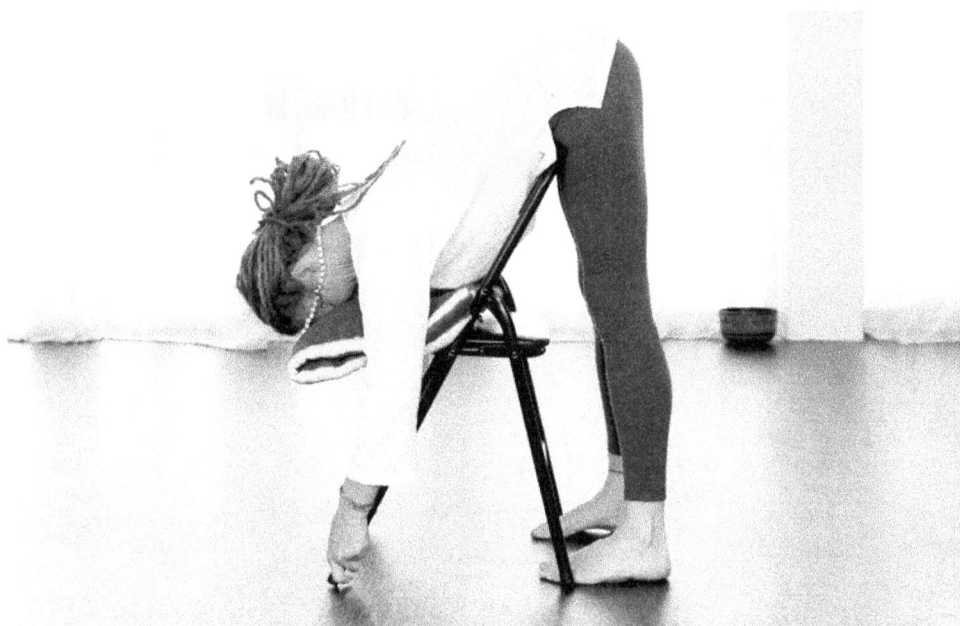

Integrate your spaces.

Supported Setu Bandha (Bridge pose):

See Week 3, page 55 and Week 5, page 93.

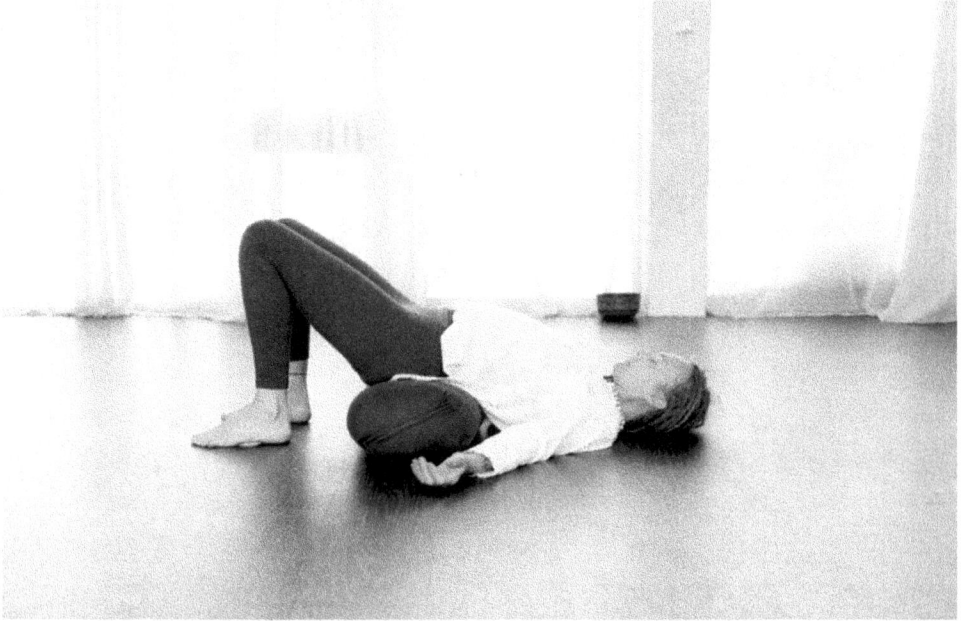

Breath it all down. **Gomukhasana (Cow face pose):**

This pose is an opportunity to simply be with what is. There's no need to challenge it or to 'try'. Just allow its winding in to bring you home to the container of the hips, your sense of centre and the deep, deep ground that calls you to its embrace.

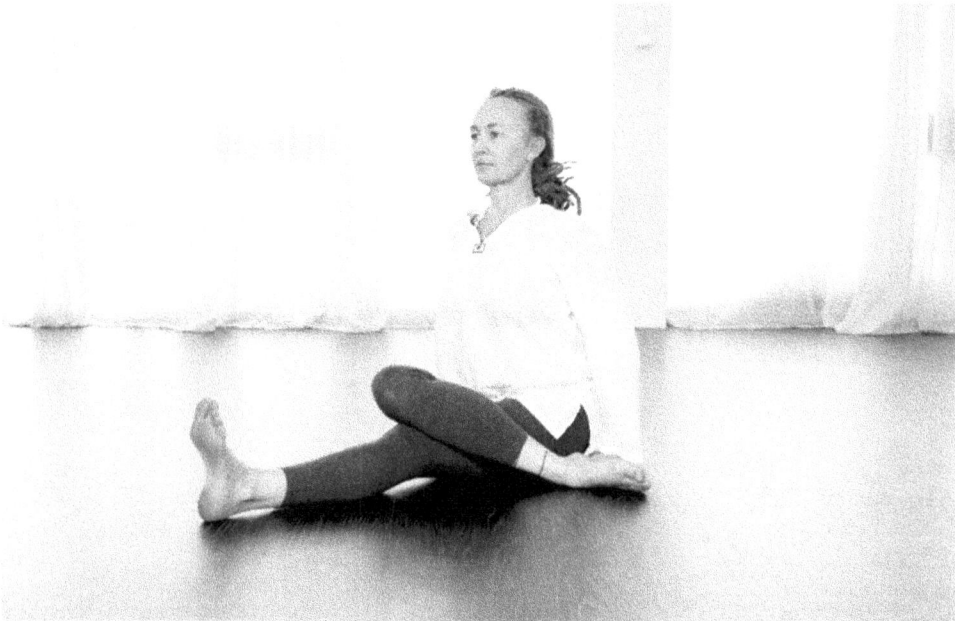

Roll up to sitting with both legs out straight in front of you.

Slide your left foot under the right knee to the outside of the right hip. Then cross your right leg over the left, stacking the right knee on top of the left, and bringing the right foot to the outside of the left hip.

Sit evenly on the sitting bones — that may mean bringing a block or blanket in to support the body.

This can be strong on the knees and outer hips. If it's too much for you, practice the single leg version by folding the right knee over the left only. In this version the left leg remains out long on the floor. Even with tight hips and knees, you should find this one accessible.

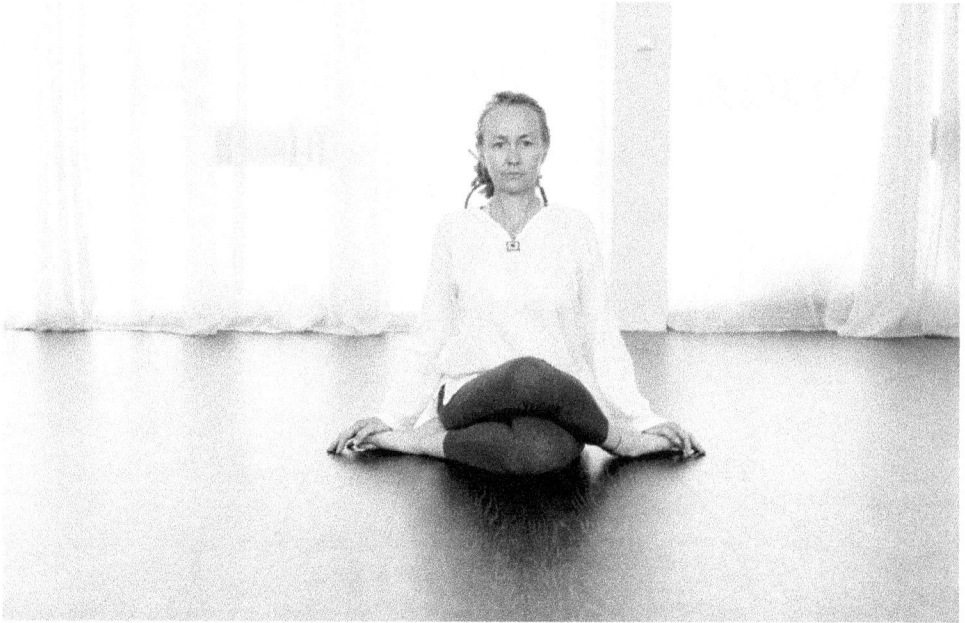

Increase the sensation of this sequence here by adding these variations.

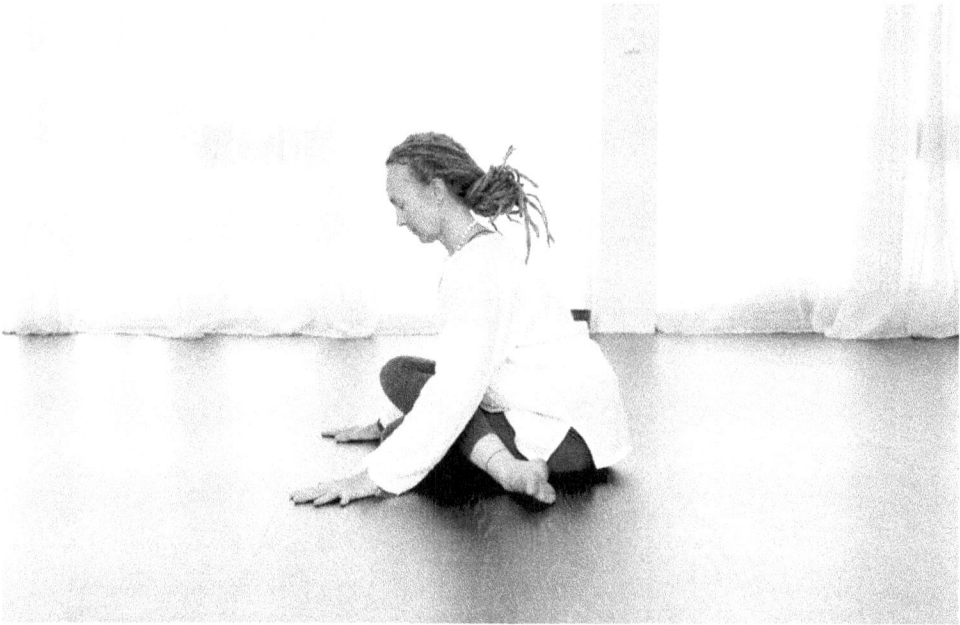

i) Exhale with your right hand to the floor outside the right hip, left arm comes over to the right in a lateral stretch.

Inhale and rise to the centre.

Exhale and repeat on the left.

Repeat 4 times.

ii) Twist to the left. Hold for 3 – 5 breaths.

iii) Forward fold for 3 – 5 breaths, relaxing the outer hips

Repeat on the opposite side.

Downward dog can feel mighty after deep folded inquiry.

Let it come home.
Supta Paschimottanasana (Reclining Forward fold):

This is the perfect place to round out a sequence that holds its intention in 'coming home'. Forward folds spiral us in, we then rebound off the inner container of that spiral to reconnect with our outer spaces in a new way, coiling back in again, renewed. Listen and be still in this shape, hold it for as long as you can with ease and fall back into all of you.

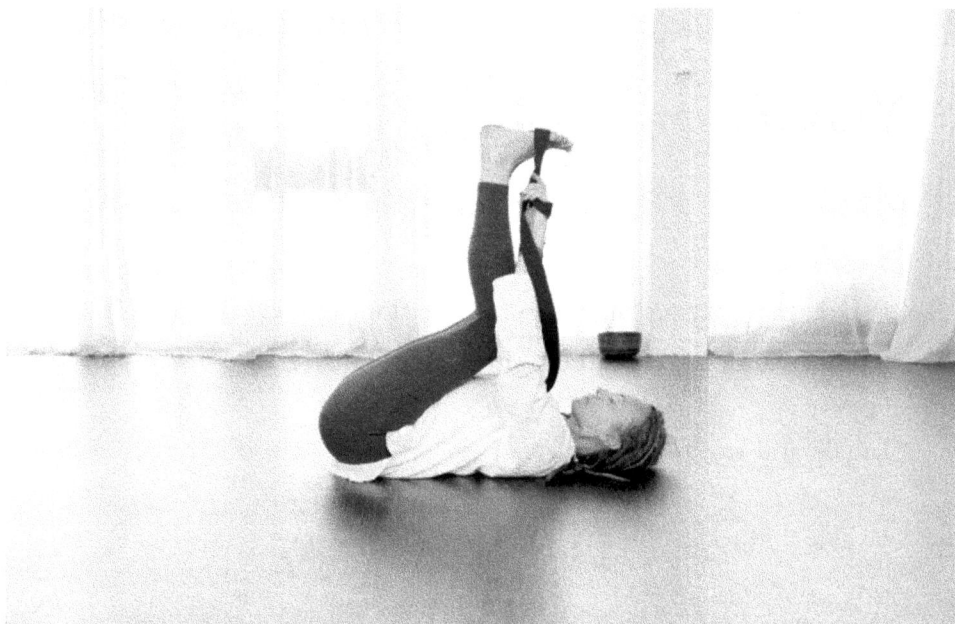

Lie on your back. Draw both knees into your chest and loop the strap around the balls of the feet.

Exhale and straighten or partially straighten the legs towards the ceiling. Shoulders, throat and forehead are soft here and the breath is long, unhurried and continuous.

In and down. **Sivasana (Rest Pose):**

3 – 5 minutes minimum.

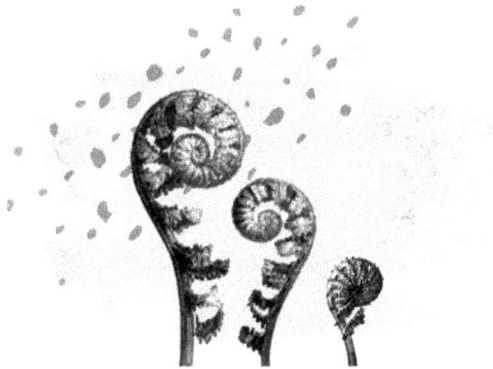

The work of the first six weeks after childbirth is a crossing of sorts. While we can read about it, look at pictures and indulge our fantasy, we can't really know it until we arrive. We are each from a mother line, a bloodline of women who have turned up for this work in their varying ways. Some of us will arrive on this new shore with endless support and extraordinary role models, others of us are empty handed. All of us are unsure, each one finding her own way, and each journey magnificent, come what may. The passage from Maiden to Mother is real and raw, celebrated throughout time as a Spiritual initiation into a profound period in your life. Its gifts hang like low fruit yet we have been taught to walk by in a hurry to return to 'normal'. During birth and the weeks immediately afterwards a door opens for a very short time to a rich and deeply profound inheritance. I hope that in some small way you have tasted that magic among these pages and found within yourself, an initiation into the powerful natural mother you are here to be.

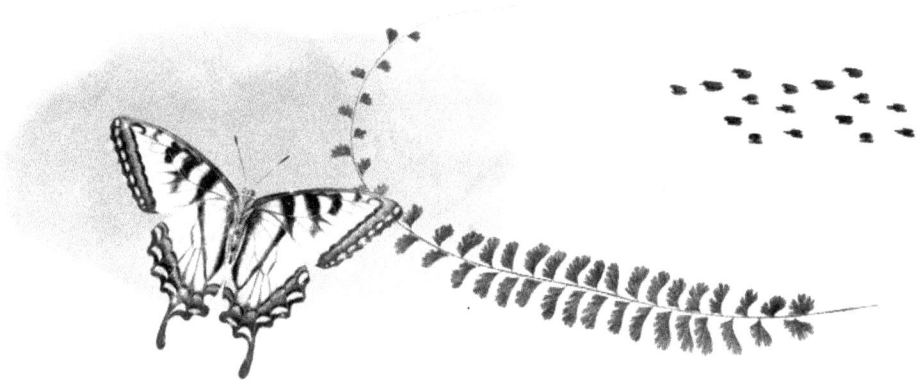

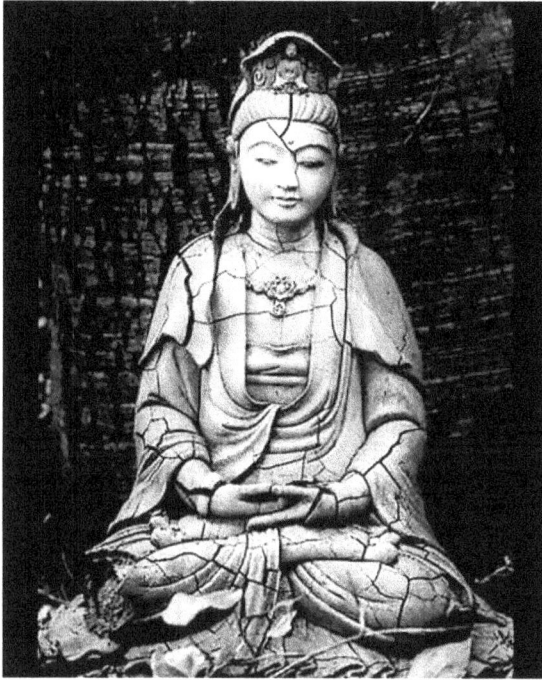

With thanks, I would like to finish this story for me, and begin it for you, in the benevolence and compassionate wisdom of Kuan Yin, Goddess of Mercy and protector of all of us as Mothers.

That she might nourish and mother you — the Mother — as you make this great life journey. That you might pass on this joy, love and selfless devotion just as it is, held in a Mother's great heart — Yours.

And that your sons and daughters grow strong and aligned within its radiant light.

Thank you and Namaste

www.ingramcontent.com/pod-product-compliance
Lightning Source LLC
Chambersburg PA
CBHW080400030426
42334CB00024B/2943